W9-BTS-737

Through the
Rocky Road
and into the
Rainbow
Sherbet

Other books by Laura Jensen Walker

*Thanks for the Mammogram!*
*Mentalpause*
*Ferris Wheels, Daffodils & Hot Fudge Sundaes*
*Dated Jekyll, Married Hyde*

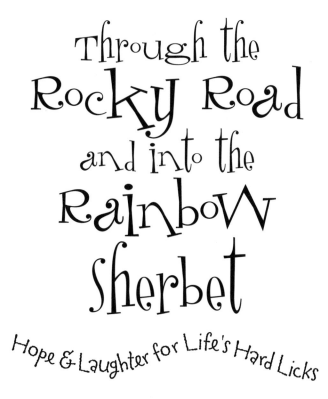

# Through the Rocky Road and into the Rainbow Sherbet

## Hope & Laughter for Life's Hard Licks

### Laura Jensen Walker

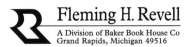

Fleming H. Revell
A Division of Baker Book House Co
Grand Rapids, Michigan 49516

Published by Fleming H. Revell
a division of Baker Book House Company
P.O. Box 6287, Grand Rapids, MI 49516-6287

Printed in the United States of America

Library of Congress Cataloging-in-Publication Data

Walker, Laura Jensen.
    Through the rocky road and into the rainbow sherbet : hope and laughter for life's hard licks / Laura Jensen Walker.
        p.    cm.
    ISBN 0-8007-5826-9 (pbk.)
    1. Christian life—Anecdotes.   I. Title.
BV4501.3 .W35  2002
248.4′02′07—dc21                                              2002004089

For current information about all releases from Baker Book House, visit our web site:
                http://www.bakerbooks.com

For my best friend, Lana,
who *loves* ice cream
and who has walked beside me down many rocky roads

And in memory of my beloved Grandpa Augie,
who always bought me ice cream

# Contents

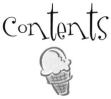

Contents

# Foreword

As you will discover when you open these pages, Laura Jensen Walker understands what it feels like to hurt. She also knows the ingredients for healing: prayer, friends, laughter, and tears—and great stories of others who've traversed life's rocky roads as well. Laura has survived a broken heart, the death of a loved one, breast cancer, and being trapped in another country on that infamous day of 2001, when America fell to her knees—in pain and prayer. She's not only survived bad hair days—but no hair days. Through it all she's discovered the truth so many of us are also realizing: God lives really close to the floor of our lives.

But how do we know he is there? That he cares? Though he sometimes shouts his love to us through megaphone experiences, mostly he comes to us in the little things. Moments of grace, one small good gift upon another. Our duty is to open our eyes and ears to receive his tender mercies.

To know Laura—in person or through her writing—is to know someone who *relishes* life. I love to be around her, to receive her e-mails, to read her chapters (which are as addicting as popcorn), because she knows how to squeeze the joy out of small things: a great quote, a fine meal, a wonderful memory, laughter at her own foibles. Life's blessings and lessons—small-sized and extra-large—are captured in her heart, penned on paper, then generously served up to us, her audience.

You are in for a treat, girlfriends. Get ready to enjoy this literary sundae of love, smothered in the whipped cream of empathy and topped off with a bright red cherry of humor. I guarantee you will feel refreshed. (And make at least one or two runs to the ice-cream store!)

Blessings to all who open these pages,

*BECKY FREEMAN*
*WWW.BECKYFREEMAN.COM*
*BEST-SELLING AUTHOR AND HUMORIST*

# Introduction

*If seeds in the black earth can turn into such beautiful*
*roses, what might not the heart of man become*
*in its long journey toward the stars?*
G. K. CHESTERTON

*I scream, you scream, we all scream for ice cream!*
UNKNOWN

I don't know anybody who doesn't love ice cream (except
maybe my lactose-intolerant editor). I've loved ice
cream ever since I was a kid and I'd stir the chocolate
syrup into my bowl of rapidly melting vanilla. I was fas-
cinated by the stripy mixture of black-and-white that
eventually became a mass of yummy swirling chocolate.

My chocolate addiction began at an early age.

Over the years, my tastebuds have expanded to encom-
pass a whole new rainbow of ice-cream flavors: strawberry
swirl, mint chocolate chip, chocolate chip cookie dough,
cookies and cream—as long as it's Oreos and not some
posturing pretender—and even rocky road. Although, I
must confess, I've never liked nuts all that well so I usually spit them out (very ladylike and discreetly, of course)
into my napkin or just leave them untouched in the bottom of the bowl.

That's kind of how I feel about the rocky parts of life. I don't like when I'm going through them, so I try to skip over them, swerve to avoid them, or spit them out altogether.

When that doesn't work, I go for laughter.

I've made a habit of using laughter to cope with the difficult things in life—breast cancer: *Thanks for the Mammogram!*; midlife and menopause: *Mentalpause*; and adjusting to those male/female marital differences: *Dated Jekyll, Married Hyde*. But the book you're reading now wound up being one of the hardest I've written as I encountered some rocky roads I didn't expect.

I was in the middle of writing this when the terrible events of September 11 occurred. Actually, I was taking a two-week break. My husband, Michael, and I were in England halfway through our vacation at the time of our national tragedy.

As much as I adore England, and as kind as the English people were to us, like everyone else, I was heartbroken, devastated, and in a state of shock.

And all I wanted was to be home.

But there were no flights out to the United States, so all we could do was carry on with our plans and wait for our return home on our scheduled flight the next week.

A couple days after the attack, we happened upon a "prayer service for America" in a centuries-old English church. Still rather shell-shocked, we stumbled inside in our jeans and knapsacks next to well-dressed Brits searching for solace. The prayers and ministerial words of comfort brought a much-needed touch of healing to our wounded, aching hearts. And when we all stood together at the end of the service and sang "Onward Christian Soldiers," we wept.

After we arrived stateside, I didn't pick up my pen for a month.

The last thing in the world I felt was funny. And the last thing in the world I wanted to do was write another funny book. I just wanted to curl up in a corner and hide.

But October is National Breast Cancer Awareness Month, and I had speaking obligations to fulfill. I did so with a heavy heart, feeling like a fraud as I told my funny stories about using humor to cope with cancer.

And then in the middle of that rocky road month, God sent me a great big marshmallow.

I had a speaking engagement for a women's cancer event, and when I arrived, the event organizer told me that after the events of September 11, they'd wondered if perhaps they shouldn't cancel the evening. Or at least change the humor focus.

But she said that in the past week or so, ticket sales had skyrocketed, and it was one of the largest turnouts they'd ever had!

It wasn't me. It was the promise of humor.

"People said they need to laugh," she told me. Upon hearing that, the heaviness in my chest lifted. And when I walked onstage that night, everyone in the audience was sporting a red clown nose. That set the tone for one great big yuks fest. Wave upon wave of healing laughter rolled over me and bathed me in a rainbow of warmth at what turned out to be the best speaking engagement I'd ever had.

It was a God thing, not a Laura thing. Thank you, Lord, for your sweet gifts when we most need them.

After that, I was able to write. And you're holding the finished product in your hands. My hope for you, sweet reader, is that this book will help you see that all of us go through rocky roads of one kind or another—some are just annoying little bumps in the road; others are huge, overwhelming boulders that we fear will crush us.

But, if we endure through them, God always has a big beautiful rainbow waiting on the other side. Besides, in the middle of our rocky road, he often sends us a nice sweet marshmallow or two to make the hard licks a little more palatable.

So, please, grab a scoop of your favorite flavor and join me.

*Consider it pure joy, my brothers,*
*whenever you face trials of many kinds,*
*because you know that the testing of your faith*
*develops perseverance.*
JAMES 1:2–3

*I pray also that the eyes of your heart*
*may be enlightened in order that you*
*may know the hope to which he has called you,*
*the riches of his glorious inheritance in the saints,*
*and his incomparably great power for us who believe.*
EPHESIANS 1:18–19

## One

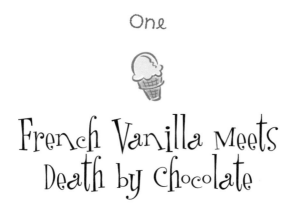

# French Vanilla Meets Death by Chocolate

How two people—sometimes even our mate—
can be as different as black and white.
But they still go really well together.

*So God created man in his own image, in the image of God*
*he created him; male and female he created them. . . . God*
*saw all that he had made, and it was very good.*
GENESIS 1:27, 31

My husband and I are soul mates.
We're in sync all the time and never have any differences.

Right.

The reality is, although Michael and I have a lot in common—we're both creative types who love Puccini, Renoir, and Jimmy Stewart and aren't really into sports (unless they're in video form like *Field of Dreams*)—our personalities are as different as French vanilla ice cream and death-by-chocolate cake.

I'm outgoing, optimistic, and talkative. I can talk to almost anyone about almost anything—save sports and science (okay, math too!)—for hours and hours. Okay, so I'm a little *too* talkative.

Michael doesn't like to just sit and talk.

He's happiest when he's doing something with his hands—whether it's painting, quilting, woodworking, or gardening. He's artistic, sensitive, and realistic, which I in my relentless optimism occasionally read as pessimistic.

Of course, that's generally when he pops one of my fantasy pie-in-the-sky bubbles.

"Honey, let's take a trip to Europe this year AND remodel the kitchen!" I'll eagerly suggest.

"Dear, we can't afford both—actually, either—with all of our bills."

Pessimist.

I'm also strong-willed, impulsive, and mercurial. I can change my mind, and focus, in seconds—a trait that has been known to drive Michael up the wall occasionally.

Like for instance when we've agreed to do a specific project for a specific room in the house so Michael drives to the hardware store and plunks down a hundred dollars for supplies. And by the time he gets home, I've already moved into another room and am knee-deep in a new project—which, of course, I expect him to help me with right then.

He says I give him whiplash.

---

## He says I give him whiplash.

---

That's because he's more thoughtful and measured. He takes his time, collects all the facts, looks at the big picture, and then sets his course of action.

I usually jump in heart—or mood—first.

That's because I'm a dreamer, first-class. Have been all my life.

Michael's a dreamer too. But since meeting me, his dreams have had to become more anchored in reality—which is a good thing or we'd probably starve.

Part of my dreaming involves decorating. I love to paint, wallpaper, swap one picture for another, and rearrange furniture.

Michael doesn't get the rearranging bit.

I tell him it's a girl thing. I come from a long line of female furniture rearrangers—of whom my mom is the queen. And having apprenticed under that master furniture rearranger, I learned my craft well and can rearrange with the best of them.

But sometimes it drives my French vanilla husband crazy.

Like when I change the living room three times in three months.

But the time I really took the death-by-chocolate cake was when I decided I needed to turn the guest room-cum-office into my office exclusively—something I desperately needed. There wasn't enough space for a desk, so I'd been using the bed as one—which wasn't very efficient, since it didn't have drawers. And the lumpy surface was kinda hard to write on.

I came up with a brilliant solution to the problem.

"Honey, I have a great idea," I announced excitedly, bouncing into his workroom one Saturday where he was busy making Christmas gifts. "Let's turn the guest room into my office and make your workroom the guest room! We can move your desk out to the garage or just get rid of it altogether since you already have a workbench out there."

I thought it was a great idea.

Michael didn't.

He said he didn't mind moving the extra bed into his room, where our infrequent guests could stay, but he wasn't about to move his big, heavy, functional (and to me, ugly) metal desk into the garage, and that was that. On this, he wouldn't budge. Usually, he budged.

"I *love* this desk," he said. "You can stand on this desk!" (although why anyone would want to is beyond me). "Besides," he added, "I need someplace in the house—*not* the garage—that's mine."

I started to pout, but before I could even finish sticking out my lower lip, he took his car keys and left, saying he wanted to give me time to think about it.

I couldn't believe it! He didn't even stay and talk through this with me. He just left.

Such a man.

I was furious!

I whined and cried and then cried and whined some more, which made me hungry and dissipated my anger.

So I cut myself a big piece of chocolate cake and added a scoop of French vanilla ice cream. As I enjoyed the texture and taste of the two flavors that went so well together, I realized Michael was right. Everybody needs their own space. And it wasn't fair to ask him to give up his only space inside and relegate him to the hot, dusty garage. As I finished my dessert, I looked around at all the possibilities and came up with a perfect plan.

When Michael came home a little nervously two hours later, he found the entire house in disarray and me rearranging furniture.

I kissed him and apologized for being such a thoughtless, selfish brat.

"And guess what, honey? I have a great idea: We'll just rearrange all the other rooms in the house so you can have your workroom, and I can have my office!"

This was one time when Michael was thankful for my ability to change my mind—and focus—in a split second.

And this time it didn't even give him whiplash.

*Submit to one another out of reverence for Christ.*
EPHESIANS 5:21

## Scoop for Thought

Some flavors are delicious by themselves,
but together, they're truly scrumptious!

Two

# The Jamoca Almond Jerk

When life jerks you around unexpectedly,
often it's God trying to get your attention.
Can you say crunch time?

*You may not realize it when it happens, but a kick in the teeth may be the best thing in the world for you.*
WALT DISNEY

The week before our wedding, my fiancé (not Michael) dumped me.

Sure, it sounds nicer to say he "called off the wedding" or "broke up with me," but beneath those pretty explanations is still the cold hard reality: I was dumped.

Talk about a rocky road.

Those of us who've been dumped know that we "dumpees" employ a host of euphemisms to explain our situation at the time of the official dumping: "We've decided to postpone the wedding a while. . . . He needs some more time. . . . We're just taking things a bit slower. . . . "

Yada, yada, yada.

Whatever spin you put on it, when it happened, I was more than devastated by this abrupt and unexpected jerk to a life I thought was finally going to be one of wedded bliss.

My heart had never hurt so much. Maybe it's because up to that point, I hadn't had a very good track record with men. Either the wrong ones were always running after me or I was chasing after the ones who didn't want to be caught.

I never was very good at sports.

This breakup was especially painful because this was a good Christian man—the man I'd counted on spending my happily ever after with.

Except he bailed before the ever after.

I met my fiancé when I was a shiny new Christian less than a week old in the Lord. He was single, Christian, and had a beard. What more could a girl ask for? Especially this girl. I'm partial to beards.

Looking back now, I clearly see God's hand in this. The man and I didn't really have too much in common:

He loved to backpack. I loved to lie back and read.

He liked melmac dishes. I liked bone china.

He was serious and quiet. I was quite the life of the party.

He was an outdoors type. I was definitely an indoors gal—which was sharply brought into focus during the episode I refer to as the "A man, a woman, and a raft" incident.

While we were dating, my fiancé invited me to go rafting down the river with him and two other couples, his best friends from college. I was a little hesitant because I'm no water baby. In fact, I'm kind of afraid of water. Plus, I don't do swimsuits in public. Something about exposing all that white flesh to the world. . . .

But my sweetheart painted a pretty picture of a picnic lunch and a lazy Saturday afternoon gliding down the river with the sun on our faces. "You won't even get wet," he promised.

Gamely, I finally agreed, donning a T-shirt, shorts (those walking-type ones that come down to the knees), and a brand-new pair of Keds.

The first clue I had that this wasn't going to be exactly the idyllic afternoon I'd envisioned came when I discovered we had to blow up our own rafts.

By mouth.

Turns out the bicycle pump he'd brought along to inflate the rafts was broken. So for a while, we each took turns huffing and puffing in the hot sun with the sweat pouring down our faces—until our friends found another pump we could use.

Quite an auspicious beginning to our day on the river.

My next rude awakening came when it was time to launch the rafts. I watched in horror from the shore as the rest of our party waded into the water and then one by one clambered into their rafts.

"C'mon," my fiancé beckoned from the water.

"You told me I wouldn't get wet," I pouted, looking down at my brand-new and very dry Keds.

I think that may have been when he first began to see the writing on the water.

It took me a lot longer. But then, I've always been stubborn. And when I want something, I want it, whether it's good for me or not.

This was further demonstrated during the sewing machine versus typewriter incident.

My fiancé had some very clear-cut ideas of what he wanted in a wife. (Don't we all? Whether it is a husband or wife?)

His list of wife-wants included:

Long hair (I was growing mine out)

Slender (I was trying to lose weight)

A college degree (I planned to get to that eventually)

A woman who could sew (I sewed once—Kathy whats-hername's finger to my muumuu in seventh-grade home ec)

Although some of the items on his list were negotiable, on this last point, he was adamant. He wanted a wife who could sew and, to ensure that, was planning to give me a sewing machine for a wedding present.

"How about a typewriter instead? I've always dreamed of being a writer," I said.

No, by golly, his wife was going to have a Singer.

I should have seen the pattern for the future, but my bobbin had slipped a stitch.

---

I should have seen
the pattern for the future,
but my bobbin had slipped a stitch.

---

*He* knew, though. God was definitely talking to him about the inappropriateness of our pairing.

So that's why my fiancé dumped me. I mean, er, called the wedding off. It simply wasn't God's will. And that was abundantly clear to him.

But it wasn't to me—then.

I was a "baby" Christian, still finding my way and so desperately eager to be loved that I was heartbroken when I was left at the altar a week before the wedding.

Now, with the hindsight of years—both chronological and in the Lord—I am more grateful than I can say.

And, believe it or not, there's even a sewing machine in my house today.

God brought me a Renaissance-man husband who cooks, paints, builds, upholsters, repairs, sings, acts . . . not only that, the man can sew!

And he brought his own sewing machine to the marriage.

*Husbands, love your wives, just as Christ*
*loved the church and gave himself up for her.*
EPHESIANS 5:25

## Scoop for Thought

Although we prefer smooth and creamy,
sometimes a little crunchy is in order to yank
us back to the path that God has chosen for us.

# Three

# Homemade or Store-Bought

Fantasies from a country-girl wannabe.
A nostalgic hungering for a sweeter, simpler time.

*Happiness resides not in possessions and not in gold, the feeling of happiness dwells in the soul.*
DEMOCRITUS

Remember that John Denver song from the '70s, "Thank God, I'm a Country Boy"? Didn't it always make you *long* to be a country girl where most things were made from scratch and very little was store-bought—including ice cream?

It sure did me.

Of course, so did watching *Little House on the Prairie*.

I'd imagine myself in my gingham or flour sack dress that Ma had made me, walking miles to school with my head protected by a calico sunbonnet, swinging my satchel of books.

Once I arrived at the one-room schoolhouse, I'd stand braid-to-braid, freckle-to-freckle with my best friend Laura Ingalls Wilder (our names are so alike we'd just HAVE to be best friends!) as we beat mean Nellie Olson in the spelling bee.

My fantasy wasn't too far-fetched.

After all, I *was* the spelling bee champ of Racine, Wisconsin. Well . . . maybe not *all* of Racine but definitely my grade school. Well . . . maybe not the *whole* school but definitely my first-grade class.

Once my best friend Laura and I returned home to our little house on the prairie, we'd do our chores, enjoy a delicious home-cooked dinner of Ma's best stew and biscuits, help with the dishes, then do our homework by oil lamp.

Afterwards, we'd clamber up the loft to our straw bed wearing our long flannel nightgowns and nightcaps where we'd giggle well into the night 'til Ma or Pa shushed us.

I remember the nighttime giggling as if it were yesterday—but it was with my country cousins, Lillie, Kathy, and Joanne, rather than Laura and Mary Ingalls.

My three country-girl cousins were the middle batch of nine children belonging to my mom's eldest sister, Lucille, and her husband, Al. They lived in a wonderful old house down a country lane.

My sister and I loved spending the night at their house.

The five of us girls would sleep crosswise on the double bed that the three middle cousins shared—with one of us always having to hold onto the edge of the bed to keep from falling out. We'd whisper and giggle about boys, lipstick, and The Monkees long into the night—until even sweet, good-natured Uncle Al hollered up the stairs at us to be quiet.

During the day, we'd pick berries, play hide-and-seek in the nearby apple orchard, or sometimes lock their brother—my cousin Henry, who was a year younger than me—in the neighbor's outhouse. (Although my cousins had indoor plumbing, it broke a lot, so we'd have to use the neighbor's outhouse.)

Those were the days.

One winter day stands out especially clear in my memory.

We'd trooped down the street to the local pond, having fun slipping and sliding across the ice in our red rubber boots, when all of a sudden (just like the young Harry Bailey in *It's a Wonderful Life*), crack! the ice broke beneath me, and I fell into the frigid water.

It wasn't Jimmy Stewart who saved me but rather Peppy, my cousins' beloved collie-mix, who gently pulled me out of the pond gasping and sputtering—and with a couple minnows swimming in my boots.

No wonder I'm not a fan of water sports.

Yet this didn't dampen my enthusiasm for the country life.

A tomboy through and through, I loved making tree forts with my cousins, jumping in piles of crunchy leaves, or sneaking apples from the orchard down the street. My Aunt Lucille always bought bushels of apples from the orchard owner—which more than made up for the few we snuck now and then, but as a kid, it was so much more fun to pick the most shiny, perfect apple we wanted from the tree ourselves. We'd also have contests for who built the best miniature outhouse. One of us—I can't remember who after all these years, but I think it was my cousin Kathy—made a really great one out of a deck of cards.

Often, we would roller-skate downstairs in the basement, since there weren't any cement sidewalks nearby to practice on. Other times, in an inspired burst of helpfulness, we'd wash and wax the dining room floor for Aunt Lucille by skating around it on rags in the wee hours of the morning. Then there was the time Uncle Al brought home an old Jeep from which he removed the engine and the wheels. We kids made it into a playhouse complete with curtains and furniture.

Now that's what you call a mobile home.

I started thinking about all this country-girl stuff recently because my friend Jan—a true country girl if I've ever met one—invited me to accompany her on a "writing retreat" to her snug little cabin in a beautiful pine forest in northern California.

My first clue that I had turned in my tomboy badge for good came when I stepped out of the car and felt my white sandals sink into the dusty dirt.

E-yew. I just hate it when my feet get dirty. Don't you?

But I bravely resisted the urge to wash them the second we entered the cabin, reminding myself that I wasn't in Kansas anymore, so I shouldn't expect a gleaming yellow brick road.

Inside the adorable cabin was a loft—just like the one where Mary and Laura Ingalls used to sleep! How exciting. Only problem was that in all my Little House dreams, I was a pigtailed little girl happily scampering up the steep ladder to the loft. . . .

I haven't been pigtailed or little in years.

And I can't recall the last time I scampered.

---

I haven't been pigtailed
or little in years.
And I can't recall the last time
I scampered.

---

Petite country-girl Jan saved the day, however, by announcing she'd sleep in the loft and I could take the downstairs guest room.

Heavy sigh of relief.

To show my gratitude, I made dinner that first night.

Okay, so it wasn't Ma Ingalls' beef stew and flaky home-made biscuits, but I'm willing to bet that my pasta with sauce from a jar and store-bought rolls could easily rival her cooking any day.

Who says I'm not a country girl?

Jan.

Especially after we tried to eat outside the second night and got swarmed by "meat bees" (that looked suspiciously like hornets to me). Jan calmly swatted them away and continued talking and eating, while I edged closer to the screen door, saying, "I think it might be a little bit cooler inside. . . . "

Later that night as we were typing away on our trusty laptops, several gnats, lured by the glow of my computer, began hovering around my face. I'd swat at them and continue typing, but pretty soon my punctuation began to get messed up. I couldn't tell if the mark on my paper was a comma or a gnat.

One more country-girl strike against me.

I simply don't like bugs (or any kind of critter—birds, bats, mosquitoes) flying in front of my face.

Which is kind of a problem in the great outdoors.

Guess I just have to face the fact that the terrible tomboy has grown into a big W.U.S.S. with a capital W (Woman Unable to Survive in the Sticks).

But I'm still not willing to concede that I'm not a country girl. I really, really do love the great outdoors and all its beauty.

As long as I can enjoy it from the comfort of my indoor armchair.

*Blissful are the simple,*
*for they shall have much peace.*
THOMAS À KEMPIS

## Scoop for Thought

Store-bought or hand-cranked, the sweet
memories are what we remember.

## Four

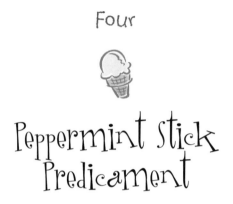

# Peppermint Stick Predicament

When you find yourself in a sticky situation,
it's always important to keep your cool.
And learn to flex a little.

*When you get into a tight place and everything goes against you, till it seems as though you could not hang on a minute longer, never give up then, for that is just the place and time that the tide will turn.*
HARRIET BEECHER STOWE

Michael and I had been longing to go to the land of bangers and mash (sausage and potatoes) ever since we'd gotten married.

I'd been a rabid Anglophile since being stationed in England more than two decades before. For years, I'd waxed lyrical to Michael about the lush green countryside, charming villages with quaint, thatch-roofed cottages, and those fabulous English accents! "Right, then, luv; care for a nice, 'ot cuppa tea?" (Must be said in a lilting, musical tone with the voice going up in pitch on the first and last words.)

Finally, after saving our pennies for a year, we converted them into pounds, brushed up on our Shakespeare, and made our way across the pond to Merrie Olde.

We arrived in beautiful Dorset where we were met by our dear English friends Pat and Dave who chauffeured us all around. To castles and tearooms, churches and pubs, *really* old houses and sweet, charming shops so that we could get acclimated to road signs, roundabouts, and riding on the wrong side of the road.

Then it was time to pick up our rental car.

Not just any car.

A silver subcompact Nissan. They call them "minis" over there for a reason.

Michael decided he should drive first.

"But, honey, don't you think I should? After all, I used to live here, and I'm much more used to driving on the wrong side of the road."

Michael was practically persuaded until I let it slip that I was driving an American car with the steering wheel on the left side.

"Dear, that was twenty years ago," he said. "Also," he added, taking his life in his hands, "your driving in the States sometimes makes me nervous. Add in a steering wheel on the wrong side of the car as well as driving on the wrong side of the road in a foreign country, and it makes me *really* nervous.

"Besides, sweetheart," he smiled at me, quickly changing gears, "Don't you think that with your, uh, little problem . . . it would be better if I drove?"

My "little problem" is that I'm directionally impaired. Have been my whole life.

I don't know north from south, east from west, latitude from longitude. I'm one of those people who happily navigates by left and right and well-known landmarks: Target, Taco Bell, the fourteen-screen Cineplex.

So even though I'd driven Her Majesty's highways—or motorways—before, Michael thought it might be better if he piloted the car. Actually, I don't think it had as much to do with my directional impairment as it did with that male hormonal need to be a pilot. It's a guy thing. Every little boy's fantasy is to fly.

Good little helpmate that I am, I grudgingly acquiesced. But if he was the pilot, this meant I had to be the navigator.

Now we were really in a predicament.

Maps make me break out in a cold sweat. There's way too many numbers on them. And numbers have never been my friend, ever since they went and stood on top of each other as fractions in the second grade.

---

*Numbers have never been my friend,
ever since they went and stood
on top of each other as fractions
in the second grade.*

---

I think it was also in the second grade that I was intro-duced to maps.

That's where I learned directions too.

I discovered that north is at the top of the map and south is at the bottom. So, to my second-grade mind, it stood to reason that north was always right in front of me, and south was behind.

I never saw any reason to change this view.

So now here I was crammed inside this teeny-tiny car in a foreign country with my gung ho pilot and a lap full of maps: a general tri-fold of the whole country; a 12" x 22", spiral-bound, a hundred-plus page English road atlas; and several individual maps with more detail. It was important for me to see the big picture (hence the tri-fold whole country map) but also to be able to zero in up close and personal on each specific area we were planning to visit (hence the individual detailed maps).

And the spiral-bound atlas? That was just because I was never comfortable without a book in my hand.

We waved cheerio to our friends and happily set out on our way.

Our first mistake came when we decided to head to Devon and Cornwall, the beautiful coastal sites of many beloved Rosamunde Pilcher novels. I'm thinking *The Shell Seekers*. Michael's thinking pirates, shipwrecks, and King Arthur's Camelot.

What neither of us is thinking is narrow roads—many of them narrower than our driveway at home *before* we widened it.

And no one has the right of way.

If two cars are driving toward each other on the same tight-squeeze stretch of road, one has to give way. This usually involves hugging the side of the road—a nice shrubbery hedge that, we soon learned, encases three- to five-foot-tall stone walls.

Haven't they ever heard of shoulders?

The locals are used to the Lilliputian roads and matchbox-sized cars. Michael, not used to either, tried to give the oncoming traffic as wide a berth as possible.

Which left me staring at bushes whizzing mere millimeters from my window.

"Honey, you're getting a little too close to the edge," I said nervously.

"Oh. Sorry, dear," he said lovingly, flashing me an apologetic smile as he made the adjustment.

Five minutes pass.

"Um, sweetheart? You're getting a little too close to the edge again."

"Okay," said a little less lovingly.

Five more minutes pass, and instead of bushes, I'm looking down a high cliff to the raging sea below.

Heart pounding and hyperventilating, "Darling, I really don't mean to bug you, but you're a bit too close to the edge."

"Okay," said curtly, with hands tightening on the wheel.

"MICHAEL! You're WAY too close to the edge!" I scream.

"Would you rather I hit the car we just passed?" my beloved barks back at me, losing his cool.

"Better than crashing off the cliff on MY side of the car!"

That's when Michael gave himself permission to lose the insurance deductible for sideswiping something.

Roundabouts are another wonderful English road convention. Rather than stop signs, intersections have a circular drive where you merge, circle, and exit—hopefully without incident.

As we approached our first one, I told Michael to turn right.

He started to exit left.

"No! Right! Right!" Now it was my turn to lose my cool.

After successfully circumventing the roundabout, Michael put on his I'm-being-ever-so-calm-and-patient voice and explained, "Honey, remember I'm dyslexic. Even in the best of circumstances, I have trouble telling right from left."

My military background mind couldn't conceive of such a thing. Of course, when Michael first met me, his manly mind couldn't conceive how I didn't know east from west, especially living in California. "The ocean's west," he'd say patiently.

"But we live *inland*," I would protest. "I can't SEE the ocean from here, so I don't see how that's supposed to help."

Now in England his voice was getting less and less ever so calm. "Right and left don't mean anything to me over here. You might as well say 'Go peppermint stick' or 'Go armadillo.' Why can't you just point?"

"How can I point when you're supposed to be keeping your eyes on the road?"

We finally agreed on "Go my way" (left) or "Go your way" (right).

No failure to communicate in our marriage.

In time, we approached another roundabout, and Michael started to head off the first exit even though I'd already told him to take the second one. "Isn't this the way we want to go?" he asked, starting to turn.

"No," I patiently replied. "We want to go west, not south."

I couldn't believe those words were coming from *my* mouth! Me, the queen of directional impairment!

But I discovered something new and exciting on this trip . . . maps. As long as I had one of those in my lap, I could make sense of any sticky navigational situation.

Maybe I should live a little recklessly and start using maps at home too.

We'd been home just under a week, and I was heading to my best friend Lana's house, which I visit frequently, seeing that she's my best friend and all.

But before pulling out of our driveway, I called Michael at work on the cell phone to ask him, "Which freeway am I supposed to take again?"

*Unless we change direction,*
*we are likely to end up where we are going.*
CHINESE PROVERB

## Scoop for Thought

Peppermint sticks don't have a choice.
We can bend. We can flex.

Five

# Cookies and Dreams

The desires of your heart don't have to be
just pie-in-the-sky.
Follow the dreams God has given you.

*Far away in the sunshine are my highest aspirations. I
may not reach them, but I can look up and see their
beauty, believe in them, and try to follow where they lead.*
LOUISA MAY ALCOTT

When I was a little girl, there were two things I dreamed
of being when I grew up.

A Broadway star or a famous writer.

I fantasized about being the next Ethel Merman or Barbra Streisand—"Curtain up! Light the lights!"— and taking the world by storm.

The closest I got was a basement band in Cleveland.

So, the Broadway star thing ain't gonna happen—something about my having no rhythm—and the "famous" part of famous writer is pretty iffy. But that no longer matters, because finally, in "middle-age" I'm doing what I love . . . AND getting paid for it!

I am truly a blessed woman. Thank you, God, for making dreams come true.

My writing dream began when I read 103 books in Miss Vopelinsky's first-grade class in Racine, Wisconsin.

That's when I knew I wanted to be a writer someday.

Actually, it began even sooner than that . . . at home in the evenings when my parents would read my sister and me stories before we went to sleep—after having our cookies and milk.

In our house, the written word was sacred.

Although we didn't have a lot of money, our home was always overflowing with books on every imaginable subject. And to help us along in our reading, my dad would drill us weekly on the vocabulary words from the "It Pays to Increase Your Word Power" page of *Reader's Digest*.

My sister and I were always reading. We looked forward all week to our Saturday trip to the library where we'd check out the maximum books allowed to one card-carrying child and then swap with each other when we finished our individual stacks.

I remember taking a flashlight to bed and reading under the covers until my mom caught me. Sometimes, I'd even come to the dinner table with a book. I really identified with the Angela Cartwright character in *The Sound of Music* who was late answering her captain-father's whistle lineup call because her nose was stuck in a book. She got in trouble for that, and so did I—it was bad manners to read at the table.

Little introvert that I was, Mom sometimes had to force me to go outside and play, because I'd much rather be curled up somewhere with a good book.

Even at family events.

Holiday dinners in our family always found the men in the living room watching football—or whatever sport was in season—while the women would cluster in the kitchen, exchanging recipes and catching up on the latest news as they prepared the holiday meal.

Exactly how much cream of mushroom soup to put in the green-bean casserole was not the most exciting of topics to me, and I hated football, so I'd always steal away to the basement or my grandma's bedroom to read. Sometimes I'd even hide under the dining room table where I lost myself in more exciting worlds—like the ones of Oliver Twist, Robinson Crusoe, or Trixie Belden.

Exactly how much cream of mushroom soup to put in the green-bean casserole was not the most exciting of topics to me.

Trixie was Racine's answer to Nancy Drew.

She was a thirteen-year-old girl sleuth, who, along with her best friend, Honey, would solve mysteries that always stumped the local adult authorities. (Since Racine was home to Western Printing where all the Trixie Belden books were printed, my aunts who worked there would bring the latest copy hot off the press.)

Like many bookworms, when I was engrossed in a good read, I tuned out everything else around me. Like ringing phones. My mom calling me to do my chores. And my little brother pounding on the bathroom door 'cause he just *had* to go.

I remember once when we were taking a family trip across the country from Wisconsin to Arizona. I'd just gotten to the part in *Little Women* when Beth dies, and by the time we got to Albuquerque, I couldn't stop crying.

We'd stopped at a restaurant for lunch, and although I tried to contain myself for the sake of decorum, I was still heavily in the grip of Jo's pain. Like most girls, I identified with the headstrong and adventurous Jo the most. The aspiring writer thing sealed it for me. Of course, her flair for the dramatic didn't hurt either. My parents tried to soothe me, but it was no use. The sobs continued. People at other tables began looking our way. My mom tried to shush me: "Laura, control yourself. It's just a book," she whispered between clenched teeth as she smiled and nodded politely at the table nearest us.

"But why'd she have to die?" I wailed. Now my younger brothers began to add their cries to the commotion. That's when the Jensen family finally left the building.

We haven't returned to Albuquerque since.

But we did move to Phoenix.

There, in my senior year in high school, I wrote for a local neighborhood paper as a "stringer" where I earned a whopping ten cents per column inch and also became the editor of my school paper. I even won an award from the American Newspaper Publishers Association!

Convinced I was going to be the next Woodward or Bernstein, upon graduating from high school I marched down to the daily newspaper with my writing "clips" proudly clasped to my flat chest, hoping to get a reporting job.

Evidently I'd watched *His Girl Friday* one too many times.

The days of copyboys—and girls—working their way up the newspaper ladder had long since passed. In the 1970s, you couldn't get hired as a reporter without a college degree in journalism or a *lot* of life experience, as the features editor kindly explained to me.

I had neither. But the editor told me I had talent and offered me a job anyway.

As a receptionist/clerk typist.

Not exactly in keeping with my starry-eyed dreams for my life. So, I turned it down, enlisted in the Air Force, and headed off into the wild blue yonder to get that much-needed life experience.

Guess what job Uncle Sam gave me?

Clerk typist.

Just the first of many detours on my path to becoming a writer. But I sure did get that life experience. (You'll learn more about that in the "Cosmopolitan Neapolitan" chapter.) And the clerk typist experience didn't hurt either. In fact, it ultimately helped tremendously in my chosen career.

After a long and circuitous route, I finally found my way back to that long-ago childhood dream God had placed in my heart: the dream of becoming a writer.

Just in time for my fortieth birthday, I received news of my first book contract.

Dreams do come true.

Take my best friend, Lana. She'd dreamed of being a teacher ever since she was a little girl: "Growing up, I always played 'school,' and I was always the teacher," she recalled fondly.

Lana "played school" all the way through college where she earned her degree in education, received a teaching certificate in special ed, and then taught for four years in the Midwest.

However, having spent her entire life living in the same state—in fact, the same Midwestern town, except for that four-year stint in college—and being in her early twenties, Lana was young and restless and needed a change.

So she shook the wheat out of her ruby slippers and left Kansas behind for the golden state of California where she hoped to find a more glamorous job and live a fun, exciting life filled with partying and good times.

With that in mind, my stylish and petite blonde friend went to cosmetology school in Southern California to become a manicurist. She learned much more than just buffing and polishing nails, however. During this same time—what was supposed to be her wild-and-crazy time in wild-and-crazy California—she began attending a nearby church and turned her life over to God.

Good-bye, wild parties. Hello, Pictionary.

Lana soon moved up to Sacramento to live with her brother while she traveled around northern California as a licensed nail technician offering acrylic nail workshops to women and selling nail products.

I went along with her once to help out but, math-impaired as I am, kept making the wrong change. Plus, I think my stubby, bitten nails cost her some sales.

Financially, it was slow going at first, and Lana realized she needed to find a second job to make ends meet. Yet this college graduate and former educator had a tough time finding work. She got so desperate she even applied for a job in a doughnut shop.

They didn't need her.

Nearly broke and breaking out in boils from the stress, she finally found a part-time job in a shoe store. Which was a good match, since Lana's the shoe queen. Before I saw her closet, I'd never seen so many shoes before—except in a picture of Dolly Parton's closet in *People* magazine.

Another plus: She got great discounts on shoes.

But she later traded in the shoe job for a more upscale position at Macy's in Men's Suits. By this time, feeling that her life was finally on the upswing, Lana—now the epitome of the California girl with her sleek blonde hair and toned golden skin—bought a new car to celebrate: a sporty red Honda CRX. Stereo cranked up and wind blowing through her beautiful blonde hair, she proudly drove home her bright new symbol of success.

The next morning, to her great embarrassment, she learned she didn't qualify for the credit financing, so she had to return the car.

That was a low point. But it was also the beginning of a wake-up call.

Lana began thinking and praying about the direction of her life. *My life is going nowhere working in retail,* she thought. *How am I serving God doing this?*

The lifelong teaching dream that she'd casually cast aside a few years earlier now beckoned. She took—and passed—the requirements to teach in California and saw a listing on the job-search board for an elementary school special education position.

Lana interviewed for the special ed slot right before Christmas. After the interview, the principal followed her out to her car and offered her the job.

It was one of the best Christmas presents she'd ever received.

She's now been teaching special ed at the same school for the past fourteen years. Lana's living out the dream— the calling—that God placed in her heart as a little girl. And loving it.

Don't you love the way God makes dreams come true?

Then there are the dreams God makes come true that you never asked for.

Take our friend Marian.

Her mom and grandmother were both teachers, so Marian determined that she was *never* going to be a teacher. She went to college and majored in drama instead, which she called "completely useless for making a living." At the same time, she was working in a dead-end job with someone who was, as she said, "functionally illiterate."

"I realized that there are people who are barely able to read a menu and they need to be educated, so I decided to get my teaching credential," Marian said.

She also vowed she'd *never* move back to Tuolumne County where she grew up.

Within a year, she was teaching at the very high school she'd graduated from.

She moved to Sacramento to pursue her master's degree, and throughout graduate school she didn't teach and really missed it.

Marian decided that she wanted a change from teaching in a public school, so she got a job at a Christian school, which she loved, but after a couple years of having "three weeks of income and four weeks of month," she couldn't afford to work there any longer and went back to teaching at a public school.

Three years later in the spring, she learned that the house next to her best friend had just gone on the market. A renter at the time, Marian had planned to spend the next two years saving up for a down payment before she even began *looking* for a house.

Praying for God's will in this situation, she stepped forward in faith. If God wanted her to have the house, he would have to open all the doors, because she didn't see *any* way she could do it on her own. She looked at the house over the weekend, found out she qualified Monday morning for a loan with no down payment, and made the offer Monday night. It was accepted Tuesday night.

Marian was thrilled to be a first-time homeowner, especially since God had flung wide all the doors!

A month later—just three days before she moved in—she was informed she wouldn't be rehired for the next school year. Then she got into a car accident. Nothing serious, but it kept her down for a couple weeks.

"God threw the house at me and said, 'Look, I'm going to provide for you,'" Marian recalled. "When I lost my job, it was like God was saying, 'Do you trust me yet? Now do you trust me?'"

Marian began putting in applications at every school in the area.

Nothing. All summer long.

Finally, one school replied—an inner-city school within one of the largest districts in town. Marian had vowed she'd *never* teach in a large district because of all the bureaucratic mumbo jumbo that would go along with it.

But she was interviewed on a Friday, called back on a Monday, and hired just four days before school started that fall.

Now she's earning more than she would have at the school that let her go.

And she loves her inner-city school—the whole colors-of-the-rainbow diversity of it.

"God has made me do everything I vowed I would never do," Marian says, laughing. "Now I tell him every day that I'm never going to get married."

> *It's kind of fun to do the impossible.*
> WALT DISNEY

## Scoop for Thought

God delights to give us the cookies-and-dreams desires of our heart. Even when we don't know yet what they are.

Six

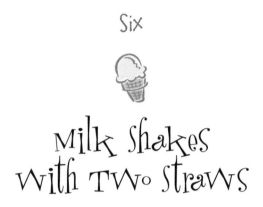

# Milk Shakes with Two Straws

Half the calories, twice the fun.
Friends help through the hard times.

*Do not keep the alabaster boxes of your love and tenderness sealed up until your friends are dead. Fill their lives with sweetness. Speak approving cheering words while their ears can hear them and while their hearts can be thrilled by them.*
HENRY WARD BEECHER

Jane Valenzuela was diagnosed with breast cancer in 1992—the same year I was.

Upon the request of our mutual oncologist, she visited me in the hospital during my first chemotherapy treatment to share her experience and to help encourage me in the difficult times that she knew lay ahead.

Jane was beautiful, bubbly, and bald.

At two chemo treatments ahead of me, she had already lost all her hair. But she hadn't lost her radiant smile, her sense of humor, her faith in God, or her determination that she was going to beat the cancer.

We swapped mastectomy stories, compared chemo notes, and proudly noted the ongoing process of our new breasts under construction. We saw each other only a few times after that and talked on the phone a mere handful of times, but we enjoyed a bosom bond (pun intended) created by our similar medical situations and shared faith in Christ.

When we did talk, we laughed sometimes, cried sometimes, got angry sometimes, and prayed every time.

It helped.

For a while we stayed in contact, but as time went on, we each resumed our separate lives—lives that included our own families, friends, work, play, and busy schedules.

And we lost touch.

Then I heard that more cancer had been discovered in Jane's body.

Now it was my turn to visit her in the hospital. She was very weak, her immune system was shot, and the medication she was taking made her tired and unable to think clearly, so I didn't stay long. Later, I heard that she had rallied and was doing much better.

That's why it came as such a terrible shock when I found out a few months later that she had died, leaving behind a husband, two children, parents, and countless others who loved her.

A couple years after her death, I had the privilege of talking to Jane's mom, Sara Dougherty, about her beloved daughter.

Jane had been raised in the church all her life and had grown up in a strong Christian home, Sara said, but when she went to college, she fell away from her faith. It wasn't until she was diagnosed with cancer that she re-embraced Christianity and rededicated her life to the Lord.

"She actually praised the Lord for giving her the cancer so that she was returned to him," said her mom. "Her mind-set was that to suffer like Christ is a privilege . . . to have a share in what he did for us."

Loving friends and family also shared in my suffering during my cancer experience. Their love and support, as well as practical help, made the ordeal so much easier to bear.

Shared experiences—like milk shakes with two straws—are so much sweeter.

Many years ago when my then-fiancé broke up with me and I felt lost and unsure of what to do or where to go, my friends Pat and Ken generously invited me to move in with them rent-free while I sorted things out and got out of debt. Becoming part of their family made it a lot easier to cope with the pain of my breakup.

Of course they forgot to tell me that this new little family arrangement included yard work. Translation: weeding and planting, raking and sweeping, and all other sorts of outdoor, getting-dirty stuff.

I didn't like getting dirty—which is pretty funny considering that as a little girl, I used to be the biggest tomboy on the block. (I think that all changed when I discovered boys.)

But now that the boy I'd wanted to marry had changed his mind, it was time for me to start getting my hands dirty again.

This extended inside as well, but not only with dusting and vacuuming. Pat decided it was also high time I learned a few things about managing my money so I wouldn't find myself in such a financial muddle again.

Practical Pat tried to show me how to set up a budget and balance my checkbook. Although that lesson didn't stick, another more important one did.

After my breakup so near to the wedding, many friends from church tried to ease my pain by saying helpful things like, "He just got cold feet; many men do. Don't worry. He'll come around." Or, "God's doing a work in him and teaching him some things; once he learns them, he'll be back."

These assurances were just what I wanted to hear, what I wanted to believe: that this was just a temporary glitch in our life together that would soon be sorted out.

So rather than moving on and beginning to heal, I clung to the hope that the man who'd made plans with me for spending the rest of our lives together would "see the light," we'd reschedule the wedding date, and things would just go back to the way they were.

But Pat knew differently.

And she knew she faced the unpleasant task of getting me to honestly face the facts. "Laura, if this was just a post-ponement, you'd still be seeing each other and having contact with one another," she said gently. "When a man is in love—especially right before he's set to get married—he wants to spend all his time with the woman he loves. It's difficult to be apart. When's the last time you saw or talked to him?"

Ouch.

Hard words to hear. But necessary. And they paved the way for my last meeting with my former fiancé where he made it abundantly clear that this was not just a post-ponement, this was for good—we wouldn't be getting back together. Ever.

Pat's painfully honest talk prepared me for that reality. If she hadn't shared those difficult truths with me, I'd have been shattered when he came for that final talk.

Those are the kinds of friends you need.

Friends who are also family are another.

Michael's sister Sheri is one of his closest friends. As his older sister (by ten years), she helped raise him: chang-ing his diapers, teaching him to swim, picking out the biggest chunks of meat in the spaghetti for him, and intro-ducing him to the wonderful world of Disney.

But most importantly, she taught him the proper way to treat a lady: "Hey! Open the door for me or I'll slug ya," she'd holler at him. "I'm a lady."

She taught him the proper way
to treat a lady: "Hey! Open the door
for me or I'll slug ya."

Thanks, Sheri, for that important etiquette lesson. I'm reaping the rewards now.

Sheri's always been there for Michael, whatever the situation, and he knows he can count on her.

The feeling's mutual.

When Sheri was preparing to get married, Michael was a senior in high school, working at a fast-food restaurant for minimum wage. Finances were always tight in their family, and there was rarely anything left over for "extras," so Michael used his small salary to pay for his big sister's wedding dress.

Six months later when Sheri was pregnant with twins and her husband, Jim, had to be out of town on business the third week of every month, Michael would stay at their house to keep her company.

"I always wondered what the neighbors thought," Michael said, laughing at the memory. "Jim would leave, and a little while later, my car would pull in."

When it was time for the twins to be born, Jim was out of town, so Michael drove Sheri to the hospital. Thinking he was the husband, the nurses invited him into the delivery room, but he quickly said, "No, no, I'm the brother. I'll wait in the waiting room." Thankfully, Jim arrived in time to see his daughters, Kari and Jennie, enter the world.

Years later, when Michael and I began dating, Sheri was the first person in his family I was introduced to—he wanted her opinion on the woman he already knew was his potential bride-to-be.

It didn't take long.

We'd gone to their house for dinner, and once I started snorting with laughter into my ice cream with Jim and the twins, I was a shoo-in.

Three months after we were married, Michael's mom passed away.

Her death wasn't unexpected, because she'd been very ill with emphysema for years, but that didn't lessen the grief her children naturally felt. And as the "baby" of the family, it was especially hard on Michael.

Sheri helped comfort him when she said, "I think Mom hung on all this time until she knew her youngest was married and taken care of, and then she was finally able to let go."

Her sharing helped ease Michael's pain and brought a touch of sweetness to his sorrow.

Thanks, Sheri.

*A true friend unbosoms freely, advises justly, assists readily, adventures boldly, takes all patiently, defends courageously, and continues a friend unchangeably.*
WILLIAM PENN

Scoop for Thought

Shared experiences—like milk shakes with two straws—are so much sweeter.

# Seven

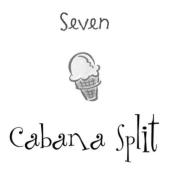

# Cabana Split

Bananas split, and so can you.
Bouncing back when the roof of your life falls in.

*Hope saves a man in the midst of misfortune.*
MENANDER

I was seizing the day long before I ever heard the words *carpe diem.*

Just call me impulsive.

Some would say reckless and impatient, but I always preferred to think of myself as fun, free-spirited, and spontaneous. I looked at life as one big adventure and was always eager to head off on a new escapade on a moment's notice.

That's why shortly after high school I joined the Air Force.

Yes, I'd enrolled in a local community college after graduating, but the idea of four more years of school, four more years of the familiar, and four more years of Phoenix was *not* my idea of fun. Life in a glamorous foreign country was!

Even though there was no guarantee I'd get stationed overseas, I decided to take my chances. And fate smiled down on me (this was in the days when I wasn't yet on a first-name basis with God). After six grueling weeks of basic training in San Antonio and four weeks of tech school in humid Biloxi, Mississippi, I was winging my way to Germany.

I must confess though, that before I began winging, there was one point in basic training when the roof of my life fell in. I was lying beneath my GI metal cot pushing and pulling the scratchy regulation green blanket through the holes of the creaky spring frame to make it taut—so I wouldn't get a demerit from my T.I. (training instructor)—when suddenly, all the indignities of the past several weeks came crashing down on me at once. I began sniffling (quietly) and screaming (also quietly and in my head), "What in the world am I doing here under this stupid bed?! I'm a smart, intelligent, and CREATIVE person! I don't belong here!"

Thankfully, that woe-is-me moment quickly receded as I remembered the old adage, "This too shall pass," along with the words of a retired veteran friend who'd told me: "Basic training is NOT the Air Force. It's just six weeks of keeping your nose clean and doing what you're told, no matter how ridiculous it may seem. Once that's finished, you get to be in the real Air Force and have fun."

He was right.

I had a lot of fun traveling all over Europe and sampling all different kinds of ice cream. After five most-of-the-time exciting years overseas, my enlistment was up, and I headed home. Thankfully, home was no longer Phoenix (valley of the scorching sun) since my family had moved to Sacramento while I was gone.

My plan was to use my GI Bill that I'd earned to go to college full-time—majoring in English or journalism since I wanted to be a writer. But I hadn't counted on the miles of government red tape I'd have to unwind to release veterans funds.

Needing cash quickly, I took a part-time waitress job in a local coffee shop where I learned how to make a mean hot fudge sundae.

As the weeks of waiting on Uncle Sam and on everyone else turned into months—summer months, which are pretty hot in Sacramento too—I decided fate must not have intended me to go to college right then, or it wouldn't have been so difficult. Therefore, this could only mean one thing . . .

I was to follow the bouncing ball dream of becoming a Broadway star. Look out, New York, here I come!

*I was to follow the bouncing ball
dream of becoming a Broadway star.
Look out, New York, here I come!*

Since I had virtually no money to speak of, I initially settled a bit north of the Big Apple. Actually, wa-a-a-y north, about thirty miles shy of the Canadian border in a small town in upstate New York, where I could live rent-free with some good friends.

I was thrilled to get a job that would showcase my talents almost immediately.

Now I was a waitress at an officers club on an air base.

Quite a step up from being a coffee shop waitress. Here I learned important life skills: like how to fold linen napkins into pretty fans, how to work a crowded banquet room with hundreds of drunken officers, and how to accidentally spill a bowl of ice cream on a too-familiar lieutenant.

I looked at this waitress stint as great material to use once I became a big musical comedy star.

After a few months, however, I realized that a small town—even in New York—wasn't going to do much to further my Broadway dream. I needed to be in the big city.

So I moved to Cleveland. A cultural mecca most people don't know about. (Seriously.)

There, I quickly secured a spot in a prestigious theater company downtown—where Tom Hanks had once honed his acting chops, no less. Now things were really starting to move.

I learned a lot about acting—behind the scenes as a clerk in the administrative offices of the company. I rubbed shoulders with serious actors—when they came in to get their checks—helped acting interns find accommodations for the season, and got free tickets to all the performances.

I also started going to auditions.

I was thrilled when I was cast in *Guys and Dolls*.

No, I didn't get the lead, but I had a pivotal walk-on role in one scene.

No lines, but the way I walked across the stage chomping my gum was crucial to the plot. I was also in the chorus for two important numbers. Granted, it wasn't with the prestigious theater company I worked for, but community theater is just as important.

Best of all, I made some new friends in the local theater scene, and five of us decided to pool our resources and share a place together. We had lots of fun in that old brownstone apartment: rehearsing dialogue, watching old movies, singing Broadway show tunes, and having loud and zany parties. One time I was the beneficiary of a case of leftover ice-cream cones from a fund-raiser ice-cream social at the theater where I worked, so my wacky roommates and I decided to have a chili-cone-carni party.

Do not try this at home. Hot chili melts cones.

One of our friends was a male model and an incredible dancer. He used to tap-dance on top of our beat-up old coffee table—just like in those old Fred Astaire or Gene Kelly movies!

Except that I was no Ginger Rogers.

I discovered this soon enough when we all auditioned for a local production of *West Side Story*. That's where I ran into a teensy problem.

I couldn't dance.

I was great with the waltz—as long as I had a strong partner to lead me—or the '70s "Color My World" shuffle-in-a-circle slow dance, but there were no waltzes or '70s slow dances in *West Side Story*. There were lots of balletic leaps and twirls and Latin mambo moves, as well as the basic musical dance step called step-ball-change, which I could never quite get the hang of. For me, it was step-change-ball, change-ball-step, or ball-change-step. (Think Lucy Ricardo in any one of the episodes where she tried to blend in with the chorus girls at Ricky's club.)

I stuck out like a sore foot. And all of my roommates, except me, were cast in the play.

I may not have been able to dance, but I sure could sing my heart out, which I did as the girl singer in a basement band.

We just never made it out of the basement.

Good-bye, New York-by-way-of-Cleveland. Hello, California.

After this dancing debacle, I bounced back with visions of writing and headed home to make those visions reality. This time I figured if I was really going to concentrate on school, I needed to be on my own in a completely new environment where I didn't know a soul.

Humboldt State University, a small liberal arts college in northern California, fit the bill perfectly. I thought.

It was a breathtakingly beautiful area of pines and redwoods and gorgeous rugged coastline. Even a non-outdoorsy woman like me would have to have been blind not to appreciate the stunning scenery.

It was a few other things that I was blind to.

Once again, I thought I could attend school full-time on my GI Bill (the concept of enough money in savings to tide me over just in case there were any complications never entered my math-challenged brain).

I started school, joyfully immersing myself in English classes where we studied Byron, Shelley, and Keats, and my personal favorite, Wordsworth. I was a big fan of his daffodils poem, having lived in England and seeing them firsthand.

In one class, the professor asked me to stay after to discuss an essay I'd written. Nervously, I approached his desk.

"Are you an upper division student?" he asked.

"N-no, I'm a freshman," I said.

"What's your major?"

"English."

"And what do you plan to do after you graduate?"

"Um, well, uh, I'd really like to be a writer someday."

He looked me square in the eye. "You already are."

He said some other nice things too; I caught words like *rich* and *fluent*, but they barely registered in my euphoric haze. A college PROFESSOR had told me I was a *writer!* Maybe my writing fantasy wasn't so pie-in-the-sky after all, and my long-ago dreams of childhood were finally on their way to coming true.

Now I really began to apply myself, even though outside of school I felt like a stranger in a strange land. But once again, the check didn't come and didn't come, and I was so pressed for cash, sprouts started tasting really good.

One day a guy I met at the local coffee shop told me about a manicurist job he knew of that was open.

"But I bite my nails," I said.

Not that kind of manicurist—he meant harvesting the marijuana from a local pot field.

"But that's illegal!" I exclaimed in white-bread horror.

He quickly rescinded the job offer.

A few days later, with stomach rumbling and just a little loose change left in my pocket, I impulsively accepted a job offer that had come out of the blue from some acquaintances. It meant quitting school and moving across the country, but, hey, it would be steady income, and I could eat cheeseburgers and drink milk shakes again.

Hunger's a great motivator.

My new employers picked me up, loaded up their U-Haul truck with all my worldly possessions—including several irreplaceable antiques from England—and we headed for Maine.

Huge mistake. Huge.

I realized it in Omaha, but toughed it out until we reached our final destination where my first GI Bill check was finally waiting. The check was just enough for me to catch a Greyhound back to Humboldt and to ship one small box of belongings home.

I had to abandon everything else.

Midterms had just ended, and I couldn't take classes again until the fall, so I started looking for a job. But in that economically depressed area, I couldn't find work anywhere—even as a clerk typist or waitress.

Broke, miserable, and alone, the roof of my free-spirited life had finally fallen in on me. How could I have gotten myself into such a huge mess? Especially when after all this time I'd finally gotten on the right track to my writing dreams.

I'd lost everything: my antiques that I'd so lovingly collected in England, a full semester of school—where I'd been earning top marks—but most importantly, my self-respect and dreams.

The only thing I gained was weight.

A friend was letting me live with her rent-free until things improved, so with the little bit of money left over from the GI Bill check, I loaded up on all the junk food I could. I grew more and more depressed, more and more overweight, and even semi-agoraphobic, not venturing out of the apartment for anything, except to make a grocery store run for more candy and ice cream.

In this rock-bottom state from which it was impossible to bounce back, I seriously contemplated suicide.

Had there been a gun nearby, I wouldn't be writing this now.

I considered taking pills, but I have a hard time swallowing even one pill, so I knew I'd never be able to down a whole bottle. Then I thought of a razor blade, but the one in my little plastic leg shaver just wouldn't come out. While I was looking for other options, the phone suddenly rang.

Mom to the rescue.

I didn't tell her what I was contemplating, but she could hear the utter defeat and despair in my voice and urged me to come home.

"You can live with us, honey," she encouraged.

"I'm twenty-seven years old! I don't want to move back in with my parents!"

"Just until you find a job and get back on your feet again. It would only be temporary."

It seemed a better alternative than the one I was considering, so I went home. In a short period of time, I'd found a secretarial job through a temp agency, bought a car, and started losing weight.

Now everything was looking up.

So how come I still felt miserable? None of these things filled the hollow emptiness inside or gave me any joy. I knew I was in big trouble when *The Sound of Music* failed to evoke any emotion at all. One of my favorite movies, it never ceased to delight and uplift me.

Not this time.

Shortly after my musical malaise, I found myself on the doorstep of my friends Pat and Ken—whom I'd known ever since we were stationed in England together. Ken was now in full-time ministry, and he and Pat were on-fire Christians, which is why I hadn't visited them in some time. I thought they'd turned into weirdos.

Listlessly, I poured out my sad tale to Pat, added in some painful elements with men from my teenage days and military years, and wound up by telling her I didn't see the point in living.

If this was life, who needed it?

But then Pat showed me the way to new life—a new beginning that only Christ could bring.

And this time, I bounced back for good. There was no need for me to split again. For the first time in my life, I had something—someone—that would never leave me, no matter what. No matter where I went, what I said, what I did, or how I looked.

And there's more sweetness and security in that than all the ice cream in the world.

*I will lead the blind by ways they have not known;*
*along unfamiliar paths I will guide them;*

*I will turn the darkness into light before them*
*and make the rough places smooth.*
ISAIAH 42:16

## Scoop for Thought

Don't make like a banana and split when things
get rough and everything seems to be falling
down all around you. Just hang on tight to
God and let him lead you.

# Eight

# One Scoop Sorrow, One Scoop Joy

Although weeping may last for the night,
a shout of joy comes in the morning.
Coping with tragedy or loss.

*Why shouldn't we go through heartbreaks?*
*Through those doorways God is opening up ways*
*of fellowship with His Son. . . . If through a broken heart*
*God can bring His purposes to pass in the world,*
*thank Him for breaking your heart.*
OSWALD CHAMBERS

When my brother Todd was little, he had a voice like Mario Lanza. (For those of you under the age of thirty, think Placido Domingo.) Such a big voice for such a little boy, we all said.

We loved to hear Todd sing and would beg him to show off his pipes at family gatherings. But he was shy, and no amount of coaxing could get him to sing in front of people. Finally, after much pleading on our parts, he'd go into Grandma Florence's bathroom off the dining room, shut the door, and sing a few notes for our pleasure. Then, overcome by shyness, he'd stop. I don't know who had the idea first—Mom, Daddy, or Grandma. But one of them thought that maybe a little inCENTive might help, so they slid a shiny new dime under the door.

Suddenly, the glorious strains of "O Sole Mio" filled the air.

Todd was a smart little kid too. He figured out pretty quickly that if we paid a dime to hear him sing, well then, surely we'd pay more.

And we did.

Pretty soon we couldn't even get a peep out of him unless we slipped a quarter beneath the door. Such a little businessman!

But Todd didn't spend the money. No, he collected it—along with bottle caps, matchbox cars, pebbles, rocks, and anything else that struck his fancy. We all said that when he grew up he'd probably become a junk dealer.

His collection habit lasted throughout his life. In his twenties, his nephew christened him "Hector the Collector."

Todd found treasures in places most people didn't bother to look—occasionally even in the dumpsters at storage units. People in a hurry to get rid of things they considered junk often left behind a gold mine for him. But he wasn't a miser, hoarding it all for himself. No, he selected things with a discriminating eye and a generous heart for that perfect item that might bring pleasure to someone else.

I still have one of the last things he gave me—silver toe taps from a pair of tap-dance shoes, because he knew how much I loved all those old Gene Kelly or Fred Astaire movies and that I'd always wanted to learn to tap myself someday.

I wore one of those taps fastened into a broochlike pin on a hat at my brother's memorial service—just a few short weeks after I'd finished my final chemo treatment for cancer.

Todd died unexpectedly at the age of thirty-two, and the voice of the boy who sang for quarters was stilled on this earth.

But I know for certain that he's singing out free and gloriously with the angels right now. (Although I wouldn't be surprised if he's also looking through the cast-off halo pile for one that might still be salvageable—even if it is a bit crooked and not as shiny as the rest.)

Todd may have been the collector in the family, but Dad was the dreamer.

And everyone said I took after him. All my life I've been told that I'm a dreamer with my head in the clouds. I get that from Dad, a fellow artist.

When I was little, I'd love to go down to the basement and watch him paint. As Dad squeezed brilliant daubs of oil onto his old wooden palette and mixed them together with his brush, he would talk to me about art, life, and the importance of pursuing my dreams.

He always told me to follow my dreams and not let anything or anyone stand in my way—especially those people who would tell me to "face reality, get your head out of the clouds, and get a nice stable job."

And although Dad dropped out of high school to join the Navy, he was a voracious reader and had a better vocabulary than anyone else I knew in our Midwestern factory town.

Dad introduced me to books, Beethoven, and Betty Grable.

---

## Dad introduced me to books, Beethoven, and Betty Grable.

---

We'd eat big bowls of ice cream and watch the late show together, and he'd reveal fascinating details about the stars. I knew more movie tidbits than any kid on the block. Still do, and it helps me trounce everyone at Silver Screen

Trivial Pursuit. For instance, did you know that Alan Ladd, the hero of the classic Western *Shane,* was so short he had to stand on a box to kiss his leading ladies? Or that Betty Grable was married to the big band trumpeter Harry James? (Although I can't remember now if that was before or after she had her famous legs insured for a million dollars.) And that John Wayne's real first name was Marion?

But even more than movies, books were our shared passion. We read of ancient cities and exotic lands and dreamed of visiting Europe someday.

But my dad never made it.

His dreams were abruptly cut short when he died of a heart attack at the age of thirty-eight.

Before my first date. My first kiss. Before he ever got the chance to walk me down the aisle. Before my first article ever ran in a newspaper. Before I won my first writing award.

Before my first book was published.

When my daddy died, my heart broke.

He was my hero. And even though I was fifteen when he passed away, I was still his Yenta Mi (Danish for "my little girl").

One dark and dreary afternoon about a month or so after his death, I was sobbing on my bed—deep, racking, tormented sobs of anguish—desperately missing my father and wondering if I'd ever see him again. I was worried too, because I wasn't sure just exactly where my father was. Dad had never been much of a churchgoer—although he and Mom always made sure we kids went—but I knew he believed in God.

Spent and dizzy from crying so long, I fell into a drowsy half-asleep state. Suddenly a shaft of light pierced the dark room. I'm not sure if it was a ray of sunlight that had slipped through a crack in the curtains or what. All I know is that there was this tiny little beam of light that spread into a larger pool of light at the foot of my bed.

As I raised my head from my soggy pillow and wiped my eyes, all at once I saw a man's face illuminated in the light—my dad's face—smiling tenderly down at me.

"Daddy!" I cried, joyously reaching out to him, but he was already gone. My disappointment didn't even have time to register, because now in place of my dad's face, I saw the radiant face of Jesus, smiling at me with shining love.

What had just moments before been absolute sorrow was now pure joy. And in that instant, I knew exactly where my daddy was and that I'd see him again someday.

Did I imagine this or did it really happen? Was it a dream? I don't know.

All I know is that when my heart was breaking under the heaviest sorrow I'd ever known and I desperately needed my father's comfort, the Father comforted me. "Weeping may remain for a night, but rejoicing comes in the morning" (Ps. 30:5).

I love how the Lord comes to us just as we are—wherever we are—and gives us exactly what we need in the moment we need it. Even if we don't yet know him personally. And although there were glimmerings of God in my life, I hadn't yet made a permanent place for him in my heart.

A few years after my dad's death, as I was about to board a plane to Germany for my first overseas assignment, my mom handed me a dog-eared parcel that bore my father's name. "This is your dad's unfinished novel," she said proudly. "Since you're going to be a writer someday, I'd like you to finish it for him."

I was dumbfounded.

I never knew my dad also wrote—I thought painting was his passion! How could I ever finish my dad's—my hero's—work of art? All I'd written so far were articles for my high school and community newspapers. I'd never even tried my hand at fiction.

I was tempted to read his manuscript on the plane but had too many other things on my mind—like going to a foreign country for the first time in my life—to read it with the full attention it deserved.

A couple weeks later, after I'd gotten settled into my new job, on a new base, in a new country, I lay back on my barracks bunk one afternoon and finally began reading my dad's novel. It was the story of a young dreamer's search for truth and beauty in the face of conventional wisdom that demanded he "get his head out of the clouds, face reality, and get a nice stable job."

The tears began to fall on my fatigues as I remembered those long-ago basement talks with my dad about life, art, and the pursuit of dreams.

This had been one of his dreams that I'd never known about.

As I continued reading, suddenly I sat bolt upright. The young dreamer was describing his visit to the ancient German city of Trier. My dad had never been to Germany!

All he knew of it was what he had read in books or seen in movies.

But I was now stationed in Germany, and just the day before, had returned from my first off-base trip to the nearby city of Trier.

In that moment, I knew that I would finish my dad's book one day.

And I will.

*Truly it is in darkness that one finds the light, so when we are in sorrow, then this light is nearest of all to us.*
MEISTER ECKHART

Scoop for Thought

Without a scoop of sorrow,
our joy wouldn't taste as sweet.

# Nine

# Tutti-Frutti, oh Cutie!

Time for recess—a sweet kid break.
They really do say—and do—the cutest things!

*The soul is healed by being with children.*
FYODOR DOSTOEVSKY

One of Michael's favorite ice-cream memories from childhood revolves around the local drugstore and their five-cents-a-scoop cones. For fifteen cents, he could get a triple scoop. Wow! There's something wonderful about ice cream that brings out the kid in all of us. So I would be remiss if I had an ice-cream book without at least one chapter on children.

Besides, I don't know about you, but after those last couple of chapters, I need something a little lighter and sweet.

When Jan Coleman and her family moved out to the country after life in the city, her two young daughters were excited to live on a farm and couldn't wait to learn how farm life worked.

The first lesson they learned was the facts of life. Among the many animals on the farm were ducks, chicken, and geese. Three pairs of geese, to be exact. As Jan was explaining the birds and the bees to her daughters, she told them that geese mate for life.

Unfortunately, one goose died.

Her girls were heartbroken. "Now what's going to happen, Mom?" they asked. "She's going to be single!"

No problem. The goose took up with a duck.

Then the goose laid a nice big egg. She warmed it and turned it, but nothing happened. She wouldn't budge, she wouldn't leave it, no matter how much the kids coaxed. She was determined to be a mother. Since goose eggs usually hatch in thirty days, after forty-five days, they all began to worry.

Jan's clever girls then had the bright idea to give the goose some eggs from their very prolific banty hen. And twenty-one days later, they hatched.

Mother goose was delighted with her new brood, never noticing that they didn't bear even the slightest resemblance to her, even down to their lack of webbed feet. A short time later, Mama Goose did what comes naturally and headed to the pond for a swim. Her brood devotedly followed Mom into the water.

Only problem is, chickens can't swim.

Splash, splash, sink, sink.

As Mama goose honked frantically and swam in circles around her rapidly sinking kids, Jan rescued the baby chicks from the water and set them on dry land. Undaunted, one immediately tried to head back to the pond again, so from then on, Jan had no choice but to segregate.

My friend Lori who lives in Southern California had to do the same thing with another water-loving creature. One day she and her husband, Marlin, decided they'd like to have Dungeness crab for dinner, so they loaded up the kids (Andrew, six, and Alyson, four) and went down to a nearby Asian market to buy one.

Alas, the market was all out of Dungeness crab, but they did have some huge king crabs in stock.

While the kids watched wide-eyed from the grocery cart, the market man gingerly lifted one of the fresh king crabs from the tank to weigh it. "It was huge," Lori recalled. "He had to practically wrestle it onto the scale."

After the clerk finished weighing the supersized shellfish, he carefully wrapped it—LIVE—in white butcher paper for Lori and Marlin and placed it in the cart away from the kids. The crab-loving couple then wandered up and down the store aisles picking up other necessary food-stuffs to the unexpected accompaniment of crackling crab paper.

Rushing through the rest of their shopping and hastily paying for their purchases, Marlin then loaded all the groceries safely in the car trunk, and the family headed home.

Four-year-old Alyson, who'd been pretty quiet up to this point, expelled a loud sigh and said, "Mommy, I really would have rather had a puppy."

Then there was the little boy whose parents believed in teaching him the correct words for everything, rather than using euphemisms or baby talk. For instance, when he had to go to the bathroom, he never said "potty" or "I have to go number one," he used the correct scientific term. One day at school, he raised his hand, and when the teacher called on him, he told her, "I have to urinate."

A few moments later, the little girl next to him raised her hand and said, "I have to myanate."

If only my little brother Todd had been able to speak similar words to my mom.

She'd put him down for a nap in his crib, and when she came to check on him a little later, he'd managed to climb out of the crib, but in the process, his dirty diaper—which had gotten a little heavy—had slipped off.

Todd demonstrated great artistic leaning as he finger painted his room with this new modern art medium. Nary a surface was left untouched—including the keyholes on his dresser. I remember this clearly because I'm the one who had to help Mom erase every trace of Todd's artistic expression.

Unfortunately, one day when my in-laws Sheri and Jim and their twin daughters, Kari and Jennie, were in church, someone had used a little artistic expression at their house as well.

When they got home, they discovered someone had broken into their house. The sliding glass door in the kitchen was broken, and there was glass all over the table. Immediately, Jim went back to his and Sheri's bedroom to check if any valuables had been stolen.

Before her mom had a chance to stop her, Kari, who was in kindergarten, went racing down the hall to the bedroom she shared with Jennie. Seconds later, a greatly relieved little girl came running back, her face wreathed in smiles.

"It's okay," Kari said, "my blanket's still there!"

The first time their parents took the girls to "big church"—rather than just Sunday school—they were three years old. Sheri kept Jennie next to her, while Jim had Kari stand by his side during the service. The girls sang songs that they already knew from Sunday school and were quite well behaved—much to Sheri's relief.

Then a hush fell over the congregation as the pastor, an impressive older man with white hair, began to walk to the pulpit.

Jennie was awestruck. She leaned over to her mother and in a loud stage whisper said, "Mommy, is that Jesus?"

Another time, Jennie approached her mom with a worried look on her face, asking, "Mommy, if Jesus is in my heart, will he eat my food?"

"No, Jennie. Jesus doesn't need to eat. Besides, he's in your heart, not your stomach."

Speaking of food, do you remember the terrible drought and famine in the '80s in Ethiopia? Our friends Curt and Peggy's younger son, Ryan, was about four at the time, and he made it his daily habit to pray for the people of Ethiopia.

Over several months' time, whenever Ryan prayed, he faithfully mentioned that country and its people.

One morning he was in the bathroom, and his mom heard him singing. As Peggy got closer to the door, she could hear that Ryan was putting the words of his prayer into song. She doesn't remember the exact words now, but his little voice earnestly singing a prayer to God for the starving Ethiopian people really touched her.

It didn't matter to him that he was sitting on the potty at the time.

Although Peggy didn't open the door and interrupt his time in his "prayer closet," she said she could just imagine his little legs swinging back and forth while he sang.

I love the stories my friends tell me about their children's views of God.

Pat was saying her young son Shane's prayers with him one night when they lived in England where her husband was stationed with the Air Force. Suddenly, Shane asked, "Mummy, is Jesus hot?"

"Is he hot? No-o-o-o, why do you ask?"

"Well, he's the sun of God, isn't he?"

Curt and Peggy led the worship at church when their sons were young. Curt would play the guitar and Peggy would sing. Ryan, who was about three at the time, longed to be just like his daddy and play his guitar and sing in front of everyone at church too.

Finally, his parents acquiesced. After all, Scripture says, "Make a joyful noise unto the Lord."

So the next Sunday, little Ryan solemnly took his children's guitar next to where his daddy stood with his grown-up guitar and played it while singing "Jesus Loves Me" in front of the congregation. Only problem was, it was one of those little windup music-box type guitars that plays a preset tune while it's wound. So there was Ryan, winding and singing one song to the accompaniment of another, without missing a beat.

No one had ever heard "Jesus Loves Me" sung to the guitar strains of "Pop Goes the Weasel" before. But that day in that church, it was beautiful music. And no one laughed. If anything, a tear or two was wiped.

---

*No one had ever heard "Jesus Loves Me" sung to the guitar strains of "Pop Goes the Weasel" before.*

---

Definitely from Ryan's parents. Probably also from God.

What is it about children and worshiping in front of the congregation?

Sheri and Janet were in charge of the sixth-grade Pioneer Girls' class at church, which meant they were also in charge of the Christmas play that year. Now they just had to cast it.

Kari, Sheri's drama-queen daughter who loved being center stage, excitedly approached her mother and said, "Mom, I want to be the angel that announces to the shepherds about Jesus being born."

Her mom tried to dissuade her, because she knew her daughter was a little weak when it came to studying and memorization, and there were so many lines the angel had to say, she was afraid it would be too much for Kari.

"Please, Mom, please? I can do it. I know I can. I already know the whole speech—exactly what they say in the Bible." Kari pestered and pestered her mother until finally Sheri took her aside from the rest of the group and said, "Okay, say the speech."

Without hesitation, Kari launched into those much-loved verses (8–14 KJV) from Luke 2:

*And there were in the same country shepherds abiding in the field, keeping watch over their flock by night. And, lo, the angel of the Lord came upon them, and the glory of the Lord shone round about them: and they were sore afraid. And the angel said unto them, Fear not: for, behold, I bring you good tidings of great joy, which shall be to all people. For unto you is born this day in the city of David a Saviour, which is Christ the Lord. And this shall be a sign unto you; Ye shall find the babe wrapped in swaddling clothes, lying in a manger. And suddenly there was with the angel a multitude of the heavenly host praising God, and saying, Glory to God in the highest, and on earth peace, good will toward men.*

Sheri's jaw dropped.

"Kari, how do you *know* that?!"

Her daughter heaved a heavy sigh, put her hands on her little hips, and patiently replied, "Mom, it's on the Charlie Brown Christmas video."

Sheri and Jim's daughters are a continual source of inspiration—and book fodder. (Thanks, girls. Remind me to give you a percentage of the royalties. Someday. . . . )

Once, her mom was trying to teach Jennie the concept of reverse values—what's important on earth is not important in heaven. "Jennie, you know how down here gold is rare and expensive and everybody wants it? Well, up in heaven, gold is everywhere, even on the streets."

"You mean we gotta *walk* up there?" Jennie said.

> *I love little children, and it is not a slight thing when*
> *they who are fresh from God, love us.*
> CHARLES DICKENS

Scoop for Thought

When things get you down, maybe it's time to take a refreshing tutti-frutti kid break.

# Ten

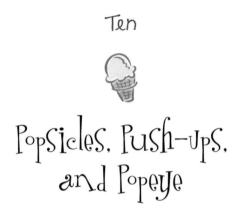

# Popsicles, Push-ups, and Popeye

A Popsicle a day keeps the tears at bay.
Flavors for every finicky palate.

*Man is what he eats.*
GERMAN PROVERB

When I was little, I was a very finicky eater.

There weren't too many vegetables I liked. I took after my dad in that respect: He didn't like broccoli, cauliflower, brussels sprouts, turnips, or almost any vegetable other than canned creamed corn or candied carrots.

But he especially hated onions. My dad never had onions on anything.

Even when we went to McDonald's and he ordered his twenty-nine-cent hamburger, he'd always be sure to specify "no onions." He'd send it back if there was even a trace of onion on the bun.

So I hated onions too.

I really liked sweets though: cake, cookies, candy, ice cream, and in the summertime, Popsicles. Especially root beer ones.

One day in an effort to get me to eat an onion, my Aunt Sharon tried to bribe me with a root beer Popsicle. "You can have a whole Popsicle if you just take a little bite of this onion," she coaxed, waving the proffered Popsicle in one hand while offering up a chunk of raw white onion in the other.

"It's really good," she encouraged me. "How do you know you don't like it if you've never tried it? Just because your dad doesn't like onions doesn't mean you don't."

It was quite the dilemma for my little mind.

I didn't want to be disloyal to my dad, and besides, I just knew onions didn't taste good! Dad had made that abundantly clear by his complete and utter refusal to even have them in our house. I think it was a texture thing. If a recipe called for onion, my mom would liberally sprinkle in onion salt instead.

But on the other hand, it was a hot summer day and I really, *really* wanted that root beer Popsicle—especially since Mom usually only let me have half a one at a time. Who knew when I'd get the opportunity to have a whole one again?

My eyes darted from the onion in one of Aunt Sharon's hands to the Popsicle in the other. Decision finally made, I grabbed the piece of onion, scrunched my eyes shut tight, popped it into my mouth, and began chewing.

---

*My eyes darted from the onion in one of Aunt Sharon's hands to the Popsicle in the other.*

---

Then I promptly threw up.

It was the most awful thing I'd ever tasted—second only to brussels sprouts. I couldn't get the icky taste out of my mouth, and I began to cry.

Aunt Sharon felt terrible. She got me a glass of water and cuddled me in her arms, cooing and wiping the tears from my face. Finally, when my sobs subsided, she gave me not one but two root beer Popsicles, much to my sister's dismay, since she only got one. Then Aunt Sharon gave us each a quarter and told us we could go down to the corner store to buy some candy.

To this day I hate raw onions.

My niece Kari feels the same way about tomatoes.

When she was a little girl, her grandma was making her a sandwich and started to put tomatoes on it. She told her grandma she didn't want any tomatoes please.

"How do you know you don't like tomatoes unless you try one?"

"I don't wanna try it; I know I don't like tomatoes," Kari said stubbornly.

"Okay, you don't have to try tomatoes, but tomorrow we're going on a little trip," her grandma said mysteriously.

The next day she took Kari to visit a tomato farm.

"I had to try *every* tomato," Kari recalled, shuddering at the memory. "Candy tomatoes, cherry tomatoes, beefsteak tomatoes . . . "

Although she didn't throw up like yours truly had with the onion, she did gag. A lot.

It must run in the family.

Kari's mother, Sheri, and her Aunt Debbie, both of whom are my husband's older sisters, thought it would be fun to play a trick on Michael when he was little. "Hey, Mike," they said, brandishing a bottle under his nose. "Doesn't this smell good?"

It did, and vanilla is still one of his favorite smells in the world. But then his sisters added, "It tastes good too. Really good. Here, try it." He did and hated it. Unlike onions or tomatoes, vanilla was never meant to be taken straight.

Another time, they offered him a drink of root beer that turned out to be maple syrup. But it was probably the mayonnaise in the peanut butter and jelly sandwich that explains why he will never, ever, eat mayo today.

That also explains why when we first got married and I wanted to tempt him with something delicious I'd concocted, he resisted when I asked him to close his eyes and open his mouth. He went for the eye closing easy enough, but there was no way he was going to open his mouth without knowing what was going into it.

I knew exactly what was going into my mouth in the first grade. My mom was trying to introduce a new green vegetable into our house one night, but it didn't look or smell very appealing on my plate.

Once she told me it was spinach, however, I was determined to eat it the same way my beloved Popeye did.

Popeye was my hero.

I sang his sailor song about being strong to the finish, did push-ups (which helped years later when I had to do ten girl push-ups to make it through basic training), and was now ready to eat spinach the same way my pipe-chewing, tattoo-sporting, Olive Oyl–loving hero did.

Cold. And straight from the can.

Mom tried to talk me out of it, but I stubbornly insisted.

It didn't pump up my arm muscles the way it did Popeye's, but something else came pumping up—clear up from my stomach.

A little onion, anyone?

Now I may not be crazy about spinach or onions, but I sure do love garlic. I love garlic the way Forrest Gump's friend Bubba loved his shrimp. Garlic bread, garlic butter, garlic salt, garlic pepper, garlic steak, garlic mashed potatoes, even baked garlic as an appetizer.

But I draw the line at garlic ice cream.

Yes, there is such a thing. Honest.

A couple hours south of Sacramento there's a town called Gilroy that's famous for its garlic. So famous, in fact, it's called "the garlic capital of the world." Every summer they hold a garlic festival. We've gone a couple times, and it's a lot of fun—especially for garlic lovers like myself. They serve garlic scampi, steak, stuffed mushrooms, and piping hot bread oozing with garlic butter. Yum.

One lick of garlic ice cream, however, was all it took to send me running for a root beer Popsicle.

*Better a meal of vegetables where there is love than a fattened calf with hatred.*
PROVERBS 15:17

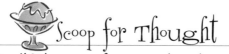

## Scoop for Thought

Don't let anyone force you to eat something— or do something—you don't like. Life's too short. And besides, you're a grown-up now. Eat what you want!

# Eleven

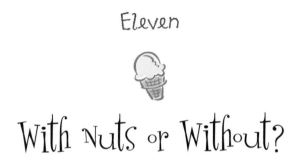

# With Nuts or Without?

Sometimes you feel like a nut; sometimes you don't. Celebrating the importance of silliness—and friends with whom we can be nutty.

*One can never speak enough of the virtues, the dangers,*
*the power of shared laughter.*
FRANCOISE SAGAN

I met my best friend Lana when she visited a home Bible study I attended. When she first walked in the door in her short red dress, blonde "tilted" hairstyle (she had one of those asymmetrical cuts that were popular in the late '80s), and long red fingernails, I thought, *This girl needs Jesus!*

Right then and there, I made it my mission to show her "the way."

After the study, I promptly cornered her in the living room where she was enjoying a bowl of ice cream, backed her up against the wall, and shared my colorful testimony with her. I wouldn't say that I bowled her over, but I definitely made an impression. I was wearing slipper socks with baggy gray sweats that bore the faint signs of a recent accident with a chocolate ice-cream cone, and my unpolished nails were ragged from that afternoon's biting session. (I was living with my friends Pat and Ken at the time—hosts of the home Bible study.)

Well, Lana already *had* Jesus—she'd become a Christian just a few weeks earlier—but she was still finding her way in this whole new world of Christianity. And I could tell that she needed my help in the dressing-for-the-Lord department.

Keeping in mind that she was a "baby" Christian and didn't know any better, I diplomatically suggested that maybe Jezebel-red wasn't the *best* color to wear to a Bible study.

111

---

Keeping in mind that she was a "baby" Christian and didn't know any better, I diplomatically suggested that maybe Jezebel-red wasn't the best color to wear to a Bible study.

---

Perhaps a nice demure floral print instead—that maybe covered her knees? And while she was at it, she might want to trim those flashy fingernails just a teensy-weensy bit, and consider going a little easier on the makeup?

This from a woman whose eyelashes hadn't seen mascara in over a month.

Thankfully, Lana didn't hold my well-meaning but INSANE suggestions against me, and she recognized the broken heart beneath the bravado.

I told her that I too once dressed in power suits and silk Dynasty-style dresses with mega–shoulder pads until I saw the light. Then I sold my collection for pennies to the dollar in favor of the standard good Christian woman's "uniform": subdued colors, demure floral dresses with lace collars—always calf- or ankle-length—and low-heeled pumps or sandals.

My former fiancé had taught me the proper Christian woman uniform code and pointed out a couple women in the congregation whose godly dressing examples he thought I should follow. He'd also taught me that since a woman's crowning glory was her hair, long hair was really more spiritual.

However, after we broke up, I began to rebel.

I chopped off all my hair (which I'd grown out in an effort to please him) in a moment of anger.

My sweet young niece ran into the same problem with a guy she once dated. (Amazing the things we'll do when we're head over heels, or infatuated.) Her ex-boyfriend also insisted that she have long hair, wouldn't allow her to wear a second modest earring in her ear, and nixed the idea of colored nail polish, other than red at Christmastime.

After their breakup, she started to become friends with a nice guy at church and, like many single women longing to be married, wondered at first if perhaps there *might* be the possibility of a romantic future. That possibility was abruptly squelched when he came up to her and said, "Don't you think your lipstick's a little too bright for church?"

My new friend Lana, "baby" Christian that she was, knew better than either me or my niece who had grown up in the church, that outward appearance didn't make the woman.

That's why they call it "freedom" in Christ.

So she encouraged me to go with her to a Friday night singles group at a large, popular, cutting-edge church in town that we'd both heard about. And neither of us was ever the same again.

Talk about freedom.

When we first walked in, we saw men with earrings (in one or both ears), a few with blue or purple Mohawks, shaved heads (most of them men), and women in leather pants or short skirts and sporting multiple safety-pin earrings. We also saw lots of jeans and T-shirts, and even a couple conservative blouses and floral print skirts. As long as certain body parts weren't exposed, the dress "code" was pretty much "anything goes."

And the music was great. One very cute guy and a guitar.

But the best part of all came when the newly married singles pastor began to teach. He spoke to us about love and acceptance and the difficulties that we as singles faced: the longing to be married, the struggle to stay pure, the sense of isolation, the need for friendship . . . and the freedom in Christ.

Lana and I looked at each other and knew that this was the place God wanted us.

After a year of faithful attendance, we were both invited to join the singles leadership group, where we headed up the social events. And boy, did we ever have the social events! Game nights, movie nights, picnics, scavenger hunts, theme potlucks, and even a huge Hawaiian luau at our house one summer.

By this time, Lana and I had moved into a two-story Mediterranean style four-bedroom house with two other single girls from church. It was a huge house, complete with swimming pool, hot tub, and a large backyard just perfect for parties. But the décor left a lot to be desired: sixties shag carpet in every hue of the rainbow—the living room was a royal-blue-and-green blend, the family room, orange-and-black, the master bath, fire-engine red, Lana's bedroom, lime green, and mine, screaming hot pink.

The tacky carpet didn't inhibit our party appetite though.

We'd have old movie nights and watch *Casablanca*, *The African Queen*, or favorite musicals like *West Side Story*. Only problem was, a couple of the guys in our group kept blocking our view as they jumped up and tried to pirouette and *grande jete* in concert with the Sharks and the Jets on-screen.

We almost lost the TV to a twirling twosome gone awry.

And the luau with more than a hundred people is still being talked about.

We wanted to roast a whole pig in a pit in the backyard but thought we might not get our rental deposit back if we dug too deep, so we settled for kahlua pork instead, slow-cooked overnight in the oven. We had a pineapple-eating contest and a hula hoop contest, and I smashed a cream pie—one in each hand—into the faces of two of the guys (which landed me sopping wet in the pool).

Or wait, did that happen at the guys' birthday party? Can't remember. Too many parties, too little memory now.

Then there was the birthday party we'll never forget.

Lana was about to turn twenty-eight, and I asked her how she wanted to celebrate the occasion. Did she want a huge potluck bash? Perhaps pizza and a movie? An ice-cream social?

None of the above.

She'd had her fill of potlucks and pizza and the same-old, same-old, and wanted something completely different for her special day. So we decided to host a formal, intimate "black-tie" dinner. Actually, it wasn't necessary that the guys wear tuxes, but some kind of tie was mandatory.

No tie, no dinner.

When Lana handed me the guest list, it consisted of six men and just one other girlfriend (who came late, so for a while, our odds were three-to-one). She'd chosen the guy she was interested in at the time, as well as the one I was interested in, even though neither had yet to return the interest. We kind of considered them our first string. Next came the second string: the two guys who were our backups in case things didn't work out with Bachelor Number Ones. And finally, the benchwarmers—on the off chance that neither Bachelor Number Ones nor Twos fell head over heels for us.

In the mood to play dress up, Lana and I both wore smart black cocktail dresses a la Doris Day, sparkly rhinestone earrings, and black stockings with the seams that go up the back. What can I say? We grew up on Doris and Cary and were in a fifties frame of mind.

Remembering our "no tie, no dinner" rule, the men did themselves proud. Every single one was sporting a tie or something vaguely resembling one around his neck. Okay, so one guy would've taken first place in the ugly tie contest with his shrieking orange-plaid polyester, and another was wearing a clip-on, but we didn't want to press our luck.

We were just glad that all the guys showed up.

The menu for the evening was beef stroganoff and Caesar salad (long before the days of salad-in-a-bag, so it was all from scratch). And for dessert, cherries jubilee.

Ooh la la.

Since we only had stoneware place settings for four, we borrowed my mom's fine china, silver, and stemware. She even graciously loaned us her best linen tablecloth and napkins. The candlelit table was gorgeous and gleaming, the food delicious, and the repartee sparkling. It was a perfect evening.

Then it happened.

Benchwarmer number one—who resisted anything formal—loudly blew his nose in my mom's linen napkin.

(If you're hearing this for the first time, Mom, don't worry; we had it dry-cleaned.)

Scratch that one from the lineup.

Actually, we never married any of those guys. Instead, God brought us the "ringer" first stringers he'd picked out for us long ago. Okay, I know I'm mixing my sports metaphors here, but they both have to do with a ball, so it works for me.

Lana and I have fun no matter what we do.

I'll never forget years ago when we went to see the movie *Ishtar* with Warren Beatty and Dustin Hoffman. We thought it was a scream and laughed our heads off in the theater.

We were the only ones. No one else even chuckled.

That film was one of the biggest bombs in movie history. When we watched it again a few months later on video, we looked at each other over bowls of chocolate ice cream—hers had nuts, mine didn't—and shrieked, "What *were* we thinking?"

*Laughter is the shortest distance between two people.*
Victor Borge

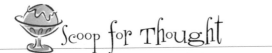

Scoop for Thought
Silliness has gotten a bad rap.
Take time to be goofy with a friend.

# Twelve

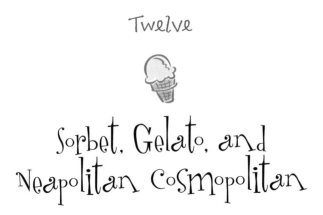

# Sorbet, Gelato, and Neapolitan Cosmopolitan

Sampling exotic and exciting tastes.
That sweet international connection.

*Don't judge a book by its cover.*
ANONYMOUS

The first time I tasted sorbet was in the summertime on the streets of Paris when I was in my early pre-Christian twenties. Yumm.

My roommate and I were walking down the rue de something-or-other busily flirting with two male American students we'd met, when suddenly a blast of air from the Metro below caused my skirt to do a whooshing Marilyn Monroe number.

With sorbet in one hand, I struggled valiantly with my other hand to right my upside-down skirt and regain at least a semblance of my dignity.

I won the skirt battle but lost the ice-cream one. *C'est la vie.* No use crying over spilled sorbet.

During the five years I was stationed in Europe, I sampled many new exciting and exotic tastes and thought myself quite the sophisticated cosmopolitan woman—a far cry from the little naïve Midwestern girl I once was. But, hey, I was acting on the express orders of the newspaper editor who'd told me to get some educational life experience.

Always one to follow orders (especially when they benefit me), I strolled along the Seine, had my picture painted in Montmartre, and climbed to the top—well, almost the top—of the Eiffel Tower.

It was with great anticipation that I visited the Louvre, eager to see the world-famous Mona Lisa.

What a letdown.

The painting was so much smaller than I'd expected, and I couldn't get close enough to really see it all that well, protected as it was under glass and in a roped-off area. Besides, from my vantage point, it didn't look any different than all the reproductions I'd seen in books and posters over the years. Disappointed, I walked away, turned a corner, and gasped at the imposing sight of another well-known but not quite as famous piece of art that I'd also seen in books and magazines over the years.

It was a majestic towering sculpture of a woman with wings and no head—titled Winged Victory—and it was absolutely glorious. We sure didn't have anything like that in Racine. I also got to see the world-renowned Venus de Milo, which was breathtaking in all its white marble beauty.

But I had to wonder, just what is it with all these sculptures of women missing arms or heads?

Just what is it with all these sculptures of women missing arms or heads?

From the Louvre, my roommate-friend Diane and I visited the nearby (and brand-new and controversial) chrome-and-glass Pompidou Centre modern art museum. Call me a Philistine, but I wasn't impressed with fifteen-foot-tall red plastic flowerpots, jagged-wire sculptures of indistinguishable objects, and floor-to-ceiling oil paintings that were just a solid mass of blue or green.

In the mood for something a little more traditional, we headed for the beautiful Sacre Couer Cathedral, which left us awestruck.

I was a little less awestruck, however, when I reached the outside steps and was promptly attacked by beggars. (Diane had already preceded me inside the cathedral.) A mother holding a crying baby approached and, through gestures at the infant's empty bottle, made it clear that she needed money for milk. Touched by her plight, I automatically reached into my purse to fish for some francs. When I looked up seconds later, a huge swarm of women and children had descended upon me, all clutching and pulling at my hands and clothes and screaming something in a language I didn't understand.

Terrified, I tried to pull away, but they wouldn't release me, even after I managed to throw some coins into the air. They kept clutching at my sleeves and tried to grab my purse. Thankfully, a cab miraculously appeared, and the driver came to my rescue, dispersing the threatening crowd who disappeared as quickly as they'd come.

Shaken, I got in the cab with Diane, who'd by now rejoined me, but I worried about the hungry children and wondered if I could have handled things differently.

The cab driver, who spoke English, explained that the hungry-baby scenario was a common ruse used on unsuspecting tourists to distract them and steal their money. It was also illegal and punishable by jail—which explained why the crowd disappeared so suddenly. "The baby probably wasn't even that woman's," he added.

Just call me gullible with a capital G.

After this frightening episode, Diane still wanted to visit Notre Dame that day. But weary, blistered, and disheartened, I'd had enough of cathedrals and sightseeing and just wanted to rest. So while she went inside to look for Quasimodo, I waited outside on the steps. Now, of course,

I could kick myself, because I passed up a chance to see one of the most beautiful cathedrals in the world. Oh well, guess I'll just have to talk Michael into taking me to Paris one of these days.

Hungry and tired, we found a little Italian—yes, Italian in Paris—restaurant nearby and decided to have a late lunch. It was about three o'clock in the afternoon, and I was feeling drowsy, so when the waiter took our order and asked if we'd like some wine, I declined and ordered a soft drink instead.

A few minutes later, he returned to our table with a champagne bucket full of ice. He set it down next to me, snapped a white linen napkin on his arm, then reached in and pulled out my bottle of soda with a flourish. *"Le Coca-Cola pour le Americain,"* he loudly announced to the whole restaurant.

No wonder I preferred Italy.

There I ate gelato and rode in a gondola in Venice—something I'd always dreamed of doing. Of course, in my dreams, there was always a tall, dark, and handsome romantic interest snuggling on the seat next to me while the gondolier serenaded us with love songs.

My two girlfriends couldn't fill the shoes of the romantic dream man, but the handsome gondolier sang with great gusto anyway, looking deep into my eyes the whole time. Although my one girlfriend insists he was looking into hers.

The other friend said he was just squinting from the sun.

In Amsterdam, I was surprised to see clusters of men squinting in store windows and pointing. Not having known many men who were big on window-shopping, I approached curiously. But the scantily clad women in the window displaying their wares sent me scurrying. I hadn't realized that the oldest profession was not only thriving but also legal in the Netherlands.

I felt more comfortable skiing in the Swiss Alps. Well, okay, I mostly snowplowed, but they sure did have great hot chocolate at the lodge.

Other fond cosmopolitan memories include tiptoeing through the tulip fields in Holland, flying a glider over the English countryside, and seeing the statue of the Little Mermaid in Copenhagen.

I also ate frog legs in Luxembourg, clotted-cream ice cream in Cornwall, and haggis (don't ask; just know that a sheep's stomach lining is involved) in Scotland.

But the closest I get to cosmopolitan dining these days is Neapolitan ice cream.

*You are what you eat.*
ANONYMOUS

Scoop for Thought

Be adventurous.
Try something new and exotic.

# Thirteen

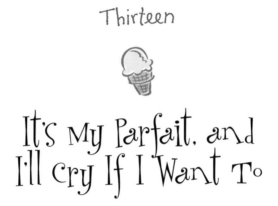

# It's My Parfait, and I'll Cry If I Want To

There are times when nothing but a good cry will do.
And we women hold the waterworks rights.

*The good are always prone to tears.*
GREEK PROVERB

Everyone told me I would cry at my wedding, but I sure didn't plan to—I was thinking more of a victory cheer.

I didn't cry when I first arrived at the church with my best friend.

I didn't cry as I got dressed in my satin Victorian-style wedding gown.

I didn't cry while my friends did my hair and makeup.

I did cry when my mom saw me in my wedding dress and told me I was beautiful.

And I cried even more when she slipped her arm around my waist and whispered in my ear, "Your dad is looking down from heaven on you today and is so proud of you."

That last one released buckets and required extensive makeup repair. After that, I vowed no more crying that day.

Michael had other plans.

We'd agreed to make up our own vows, and writer that I am, I had labored over mine, choosing just the right words, just the right tone, and just the right length. Even then, I was still editing them at the last minute. I pulled from my long satin wedding glove a small piece of paper folded into eighths and covered with crossed-out lines.

As I faced my beloved, I told him how grateful I was for the gift God had given me in him and how thankful I was that he understood and encouraged my dreams, pledging to likewise encourage him in his. I promised to love him and put him before everyone else—family and friends— because he was my lifelong companion. Then I thanked him for loving me through *all* my moods and vowed that whither he wentest, I'd went too.

## I thanked him for loving me through all my moods and vowed that whither he wentest, I'd went too.

Now it was Michael's turn.

I looked at him expectantly as the pastor handed him the microphone. Suddenly, behind me, I heard my sister-in-law play a few chords on the piano. *Oh, no, I thought, she's coming in at the wrong time! She's not supposed to play until we take communion and light the unity candle!* But then I recognized the song, and Michael surprised me—and everyone else—by starting to sing his vows.

He sang that he would always love me, he would never leave me, and that he was always strong when I was beside him. He promised to always fight for my honor, to be my hero, and to take me to his castle far away.

So much for not crying.

It wasn't just me. Over Michael's shoulder, I noticed his best man, brother Bob, wiping his eyes, and behind me, I could hear all my bridesmaids sniffling. From there, it spread into the congregation until pretty soon there was a cacophony of sniffling throughout the entire church.

Now that's what I call a crying party.

When Jan and Carl got married, they had a smaller, more intimate crying party when he took her to Europe a couple months later for an enchanted honeymoon tour by train.

They flew into Switzerland and looked for Heidi in the Alps, but not finding the Swiss miss and getting a little hoarse from all the yodeling, they then took the train down to Rome. Amidst the pasta and pizza they met some student backpackers who told them about five tiny but charming seafront villages strung along the Mediterranean coast. The adventurous couple decided to check it out and stopped at the first village of Riomaggiore.

They'd been told all they had to do was find Mama Rosa's and they could bunk there for the night. Mama Rosa was friendly and cheap, which was an important consideration on their budget honeymoon.

But, also popular.

She had no room in the rosa.

The tourist information office with all the lodging information was already closed for the day, but Mama Rosa told the intrepid travelers to call Lorenzo something-or-other, and he would "fixa you up."

Lorenzo spoke little English but knew enough to escort them through tiny streets and alleys to a cluster of amber-colored flats jumbled on top of each other. Jan and Carl followed Lorenzo up the creaky stairs and down the corridor past several doors until he finally stopped in front of one, proudly presented them with a large, old-fashioned key, took their lira, and left.

Hastily dropping off their backpacks at the flat, the happy honeymooners spent the rest of the day exploring the panoramic Mediterranean coastline as they walked hand in hand from idyllic village to village. When they finally returned to their sleepy village, it was 11:00 P.M., and they didn't know where their flat was.

So eager to be on their way exploring earlier in the day, neither one had paid attention to which flat Lorenzo-the-landlord had led them to. Now, in the dark, they all looked identical. The tired couple wandered around for nearly an hour, quietly trying their key—the large old-fashioned key with no name or lettering on it—in various doors.

"Don't worry, sweetie, we'll find it," Carl assured a weary Jan.

They didn't.

That's when Jan began to cry. And blame her not-quite-so-new-any-longer husband.

"You mean YOU didn't get the guy's number? What's his last name? We don't know that either? I can't believe this!" Frustrated and exhausted, she finally crouched down in the corner and wailed, "I'll just sleep right here. It's cold. I'm tired, and the whole town's asleep."

Carl, the cool and unflappable, scratched his head and said, "There must be a way." Suddenly, his face lit up, and he grabbed Jan's hand. He led her up and down and round and around the dark streets until they finally found the only place in town with lights on—the local bar where the regulars were enjoying their vino. The weary couple (who didn't speak any Italian other than *s'cusi* and *prego*—which I always thought was a sauce but evidently means please) held up the key and gestured.

The bartender looked at them blankly. Finally, the moon hit his eye and comprehension gleamed. "No problemo." He picked up the phone, dialed a number, and said something in rapid Italian. Within minutes, Landlord Lorenzo appeared and ushered the tired twosome to the right flat.

Ah, that's *amoré*.

Michael and I weren't much in the mood for amore after our very first day of driving together in England on the wrong side of narrow winding roads in a subcompact car with the steering wheel on the right side.

Can you say stretched nerves? Frayed tempers? Marital discord?

And to add a cherry on top of it all, rumbling and grumbling empty stomachs by the time we finally arrived in the coastal town of Dartmouth that evening.

All we wanted was food, a hot bath, and a place to lay our splitting heads for the night.

Michael drove through cramped one-lane city streets looking for any hotels, B&Bs, or even hostels, but there were none to be found. After half an hour of fruitless searching, I finally spotted a small B&B sign on the front of an elegant, slender, coral-colored building wedged between a host of other slender elegant buildings on a not-so-slender hill overlooking the sea.

"Stop the car!" I yelled.

Michael slammed on the brakes, afraid he'd been about to sideswipe a teacart.

Giving me a look that was anything but romantic, my sweetheart gingerly extricated himself from our bulging-with-luggage-and-presents car and walked across the street to ring the bell on the B&B door.

He rang.

And rang.

And rang. Then he tried knocking. And knocking. And knocking. To no avail. No one answered, and it was only 5:00 in the evening.

By this point, Michael had had enough of driving—and so had I—so he found a parking place, and we decided to continue our quest for the Holy Grail of beds on foot.

After a few blocks, we spotted a pub sign over an outdoor patio of locals laughing and drinking something besides afternoon tea. Happily, we also discovered that the pub had an inexpensive room and bath to rent for the night.

Our relief was short-lived.

As the barman inserted the key in the lock of the heavy wooden door that led upstairs, it wouldn't open. He tried several keys as Michael and I exchanged "Now what?" glances, but none worked.

"'ang on a minute," he said cheerfully as he left to (we assumed) get the right key.

A couple minutes later we heard feet pounding down the stairs on the other side of the locked door. It swung open to reveal our smiling publican. "Right then, 'ere we go," he said, turning and leading us upstairs.

With visions of being trapped in the attic with no way out, we followed him uncertainly up the steep, creaking stairs. But the minute I saw the lumpy bed, wrinkled sheets, and none-too-sparkling bathroom, we politely excused ourselves, suddenly remembering something important we'd left in the car.

After this narrow lodging escape, we decided to just bite the travel-budget bullet and pay whatever was necessary to get a clean room for the night.

At last, we found a beautiful, gleaming—and incredibly expensive looking—waterfront hotel. We entered the lovely lobby and groaned in pleasure as our tired feet sank into a soft bed of plush carpet whilst our ravenous noses caught a whiff of roast duck.

Unfortunately, there was no room in the inn. They were booked solid for the night.

I began to cry. Discreetly, of course. (I kept the racking sobs to a minimum and only wiped my nose on my sleeve once.) After all, we were in the land of the stiff upper lip.

Michael had no qualms at all about not maintaining a stiff upper lip. He's from California where men aren't afraid to express their feelings. So he articulately expressed those hungry, tired, and at the end of his driving-on-the-wrong-side-of-the-road rope feelings.

The innkeeper quickly suggested some nearby alternatives, but on our way back to the car, we bumped into another B&B we hadn't seen earlier. The room we rented was beautifully decorated with pretty peach and sage-green wallpaper, had a wonderful view of the town and the sea, and best of all, cost half the amount of the swanky seaside hotel.

We got a bite to eat, a little ice cream for dessert, and then tumbled into bed too tired to take a bath.

The next day we learned that Tourist Information would make reservations for us for a small fee.

A pound of prevention and leave the crying to them.

*You turned my wailing into dancing;*
*you removed my sackcloth*
*and clothed me with joy.*
Psalm 30:11

Scoop for Thought

Crying's good for the soul. So don't be afraid to release those waterworks!

## Fourteen

# The Good Humor Man

Attitude is everything.
No matter what the situation, good humor makes
everything bearable.

*Good humor makes all things tolerable.*
HENRY WARD BEECHER

The sound of the ice-cream truck coming down the street was unmistakable. No matter whether we were outside playing or inside doing chores, the moment we heard that loud, cheerful music, all of us neighborhood kids would pour out of our houses and run to catch up with the Good Humor man.

With our precious nickels and dimes clutched tightly in our fists, we'd peer wide-eyed inside his rainbow-colored truck, unable to decide between all the precious choices gleaming inside the frozen ice chest.

Our moms had given us careful instructions; only one treat was allowed. Which was why it was even more important to make the right choice.

Decisions, decisions.

Would it be a fudgesicle today with all that yummy, creamy chocolate to lick? Or maybe an ice-cold Popsicle in a rainbow of flavors? Grape? Cherry? Root beer? Orange? Or would we try for the best of both worlds and buy a creamsicle instead with its yummy icy orange outer shell deliciously wrapped around the soft, creamy vanilla ice cream inside? Yumm. There's nothing quite like the taste explosion on your tongue when you lick a swirl of the inner and outer shell together.

Of course, there was always a drumstick too, which provided dark soft-shell chocolate, vanilla ice cream, and a cookie cone to boot. I rarely chose this one because I didn't like the nuts on top. Although, sometimes the temptation of the other three flavors together was too hard to resist, so I just spat out the nuts.

Sometimes I'd choose an ice-cream sandwich 'cause that way I got both ice cream and a chocolate cookie! Years later, a girlfriend told me that her engineer brother theorizes that ice-cream sandwiches are the most perfectly engineered snack. The cookie on the outside insulates the ice cream on the inside, it doesn't get on your fingers, and it's the right shape to hold in your hand when you're driving.

All I knew was that it tasted yummy.

And loving chocolate as I did even way back then, I usually opted for either an ice-cream sandwich or a fudgesicle.

The ice-cream man was always in a good humor. He'd tell us knock-knock jokes or make up silly songs and sing them to us—like "Do you know the ice-cream man, the ice-cream man, the ice-cream man?" He was never bad tempered or impatient with us, knowing full well that the right frozen selection was a matter of grave importance.

The ice-cream man was always
in a good humor.

Occasionally, when all the other kids had gone, and it was just my sister and me left at the truck, still trying to make up our minds between a fudgesicle or a Popsicle, he'd suddenly exclaim, "Hey, whaddya know! I've got a Popsicle here that's a little bit crushed. I can't sell damaged merchandise to my customers . . . guess I'm just gonna have to throw it away. Unless, of course, you might know someone who would be willing to share it with someone else?" he asked. "Like maybe her sister?"

Wide-eyed, we'd chorus, "We do! That's us! We're sisters!"

"Okay, just as long as you remember to share." Thrilled by having the difficult decision taken out of our hands, we'd plop down our grubby nickels for a fudgesicle a piece, then greedily split the crushed Popsicle. Then the Good Humor man would shut the freezer door, start up his rainbow truck, and drive off down the street with happy music blaring.

I try to maintain a good humor—or at least, sense of humor—most of the time. But midlife and mentalpause sometimes gets in the way.

Head back to England again with Michael and me now. After landing at Heathrow Airport, we boarded the tube for the train station. I'd ridden the London Underground regularly when I lived there before, but I didn't remember it being quite this hot.

Or crowded.

I liked fish and chips but not sardines.

Plus, it was an unseasonably warm autumn day, and we'd dressed for what we thought would be the London fog and drizzle so we were a trifle warm.

Since there were no empty seats, Michael and I were both left standing and hanging on to metal poles across the car from each other with our suitcases wedged between our feet. It was so crowded that Michael couldn't even stand fully erect. He wound up leaning more and more over the luggage until he was nearly bent perpendicular.

As more and more people boarded at each stop and very few got off, our car grew warmer and warmer. And I grew more glistening and glowing, while my husband, who tends to be a bit claustrophobic, grew a little bug-eyed.

"Is it hot in here, or is it just me?" I asked Michael, furiously fanning myself with a tube schedule while trying to maintain my awkward balance with the other. Finally, at the next stop, a woman got up from her seat to disembark, and I raced a skinny, black-leather-jacketed teen to the now empty seat.

Although I had thirty years and probably a good forty pounds on him, I won.

You don't mess with a woman in menopause.

The other thing that had changed in the twenty years since I'd last ridden the Underground was that the seats had gotten smaller. Can you say "Laura's spilling out all over?" right into the seat next to me where a very proper English gentleman was reading his *London Times*.

But being a well-bred, stiff-upper-lipped English gent, he never said a word.

I did though. To Michael. With my eyes.

I felt a monster hot flash bubbling up ready to erupt at any second. Unwilling to strip on public transportation in a foreign country and risk arrest, or worse yet, be considered an ugly American, I abruptly stood up. My beloved, who by now knew all the familiar signs—red face, drenched hair, rapidly fanning hand motions—joined me as we politely pushed and shoved our way through the crowded car. "Excuse me. Pardon me. Excuse me. Pardon me."

We leapt off at the next stop and lugged our what-by-now-felt-like-they-weighed-a-ton luggage up several labyrinthine flights of stairs before finally escaping into the light and fresh air.

Freedom! (said in a Scottish accent like Mel Gibson in *Braveheart*).

We hailed a London taxicab—one of those wonderful great big black behemoths that looks like something from the '30s—and asked him to take us to Waterloo Station.

"Can you turn on the air-conditioning, please?" I asked the cabbie politely.

"'Cor, luv," he cackled, "we got no need for air-conditioning over 'ere."

That's when my good humor melted all over the place.

*Humor is mankind's greatest blessing.*
MARK TWAIN

Scoop for Thought

Good humor is good medicine.

## Fifteen

# Turning Drudgesicles into Dreamsicles

Just because you're stuck on a stick doesn't mean
you have to be a stick-in-the-mud.
Rise above your circumstances.

*Your talent is God's gift to you. What you do with it is*
*your gift back to God.*
LEO BUSCAGLIA

At the age of thirty, I was stuck in a rut.

I had a nice, well-paying job as the joint secretary to both the president and marketing manager of a prestigious insurance company, wore '80s power suits, frequently ate lunch at expensive restaurants, and lived in a nice apartment with a great roommate.

But, truth be told, I was restless, discontented, and bored out of my skull.

Sure, I typed a hundred words a minute, had the fastest filing hand in the West, and set up swanky events with upscale caterers, but it just wasn't satisfying. I knew that there had to be something better, something different. Something that made my heart go pitty-pat. (Besides the latest flavor-of-the-month crush at my church singles group.)

There was.

But it would involve risk, drastic changes to my lifestyle, and math.

Through a supernatural series of events, God made it abundantly clear to me that I was to return to college full-time and get my degree.

I fought and kicked for a while about it, because as you well know by now, I'd been down that road several times before and could never manage to stay on it all the way to the end. But I've learned that when God lets me know he wants me to do something, it's best (for me and everyone else around me) to just listen and obey.

So I quit my well-paying but by-now-drudge job and returned to the uncertain realm of starving student. Scared stiff that I was going to blow it yet again.

But you know what? I didn't.

My first semester back at school, I took a beginning journalism class where I rediscovered my lost love—writing. From then on, there was no stopping me. God started flinging open doors left and right: I began writing for the school paper, winning scholarships and writing contests, and became the editor of the school paper.

School was a dream I'd been longing to see come true for many years, but the timing had just never been right. I hadn't been ready. But now it was, and I was. And my college days were all the richer and sweeter for it.

I loved school, every one of my classes, except math. For a time it looked as if I might not be able to graduate thanks to that old nemesis of mine, but God was gracious, and my very last semester guided me to a wonderful teacher who finally got me through fractions, percentages, and algebra—even giving me a B in the process!

I think the hundred bucks I slipped her helped.

Out of college and back in the real world, I experienced one of the most tedious jobs I ever had. Typing in ads for a local real estate "magazine." One of those freebies you can pick up from racks in front of most grocery stores.

All day long I'd sit in my chair in the middle of a row with ten other people inside this ugly industrial warehouse and type in two- or three-line ads submitted from hand-scrawled realtor notes:

### Cozy and Cute
Cozy 2 bdrm, 1 ba bglw in nice est nbhd. Live
Oaks, a/c, frsh pnt in/out. Needs a little TLC. $99,000

### Dream House
Lrg 4 bdrm, 2½ ba on ½ acre in dsrbl nbhd. 3000
sf, Ch/a, hdwd flrs, Corian in kit, jac in mstr ba, grt rm,
frml dr, hm ofc, huge yd w/pool, beaut ldnscp. $450K

That cozy, two-bedroom, one-bath bungalow in a nice
established neighborhood sounds pretty adorable, doesn't
it? Hah! Translation: small (probably less than nine hundred square feet), old, and falling apart in a not very good
neighborhood. Especially for that price in California. The
large four-bedroom on half an acre of beautifully land-
scaped land complete with hardwood floors, Corian coun-
tertops in the kitchen, and a Jacuzzi in the master bath,
however, was a luxurious home in a prestigious neighborhood for the crème-de-la-crème—which meant none
of us working in that office.

There was nothing crème-de-la-crème about the place
we worked. The "lunch room" for nearly fifty people had
one wobbly table that four, maybe five people could sit
around, a small dorm-sized refrigerator, and a lone, ancient
microwave that hadn't been cleaned in months.

We had a half hour for lunch and had to punch in and
out. If we were two minutes late, our pay was docked.
There was a long list of rules for everything from bathroom use to the specific abbreviations we were to follow
to the letter when typing our ads.

For some reason, I kept transposing the letters for bedroom (bdrm) to brdm.

Must have been Freudian for how I felt about the job.

I kept trying to find a bright spot in all this dim Dickensian drudgery, but it wasn't easy.

Finally, hurrah! I discovered that one of my coworkers was also a big Academy Awards nut just like me, so we got permission to set up an office contest, complete with sparkly ballots and prizes to predict the winners.

I won a prize.

And soon I won an even better prize. I got to quit for a dreamsicle reporting job.

Michael's dreamsicle job was doing Christian theater. Before he got to do that, though, he held a drudgesicle position in the formal-wear department of an upscale store.

Early in high school he realized that Christian theater was his calling, so after he graduated from college, he auditioned for several companies—four of which offered him a spot in their troupe.

He selected a Christian theater in the Southwest where he was thrilled to become part of a working community of theater people. The smell of the greasepaint, the roar of the crowd . . . Michael loved nearly every aspect of working in such a creative, artistic, and energetic environment.

He wore many hats: actor, singer, stage manager, set builder, prop maker, and several office administrative jobs.

Early on, however, he realized that his job was not conducive to relationships with the opposite sex. He dated one woman for a little while but recognized that, during a busy theater season, things got so frenetic you often had to choose whether to eat or sleep. Therefore, phone calls to chitchat were frequently forgotten. The woman he was seeing didn't understand when an entire week would go by and he wouldn't call.

Can you say death knell for any relationship?

Michael realized how right she was and decided not to date again until after he left the company. He loved his job. It was fulfilling, challenging, and artistically stimulating. But after five years, he grew tired of the low pay and lack of social life and decided it was time to start a new career in the "real world."

Unexpectedly, a new dreamsicle opportunity came his way.

While chatting on the phone with a college friend one day during his job hunt, he learned of an open stage management position on the same cruise ship where his friend worked—at twice the pay he was earning in his acting career.

Eleven days later, he was on an airplane to Greece to meet the ship and begin a brand-new life. (It would take another book to share the miracles God did to get him there that quickly.)

Michael operated lights and sound for live shows, ran the onboard TV studio, and showed movies in the ship's theater. (He wound up seeing—or rather, hearing—*Field of Dreams* so many times he can still recite much of the dialogue by heart.)

He circumnavigated the Mediterranean and into the then Soviet Union cities of Odessa and Yalta. Hung out with the Sphinx and went inside a pyramid. Followed a path through people's backyards to reach the Parthenon in Athens. Sat in THE theater at Ephesus and read the Scriptures about Paul and Demetrius the silversmith. Ate real Italian pizza and got to speak his limited Spanish in its native land.

He crossed the Atlantic, crisscrossed the Caribbean, cruised fifteen hundred miles up the Amazon River, and sailed through the Panama Canal on Christmas Day 1989, which was a day or so after the canal reopened after the coup. Soldiers with submachine guns, helicopters flying overhead, and Michael hanging out on deck in shorts and a polo shirt.

Soldiers with submachine guns, helicopters flying overhead, and Michael hanging out on deck in shorts and a polo shirt.

It was an exciting season in his life filled with treasured memories, but he missed the fellowship of a church family. He decided that when the ship dropped him off in San Francisco he was meant to come the remaining ninety miles home to Sacramento, rather than return to Texas. Houston to Sacramento is about nineteen hundred miles as the crow flies. Sometimes the journey God would have us take is a little longer.

The woman God had handpicked for Michael was waiting impatiently.

Yours truly.

Less than a year later, we met. He swept me off my feet, we married, he got the stable well-paying job that allowed me the freedom to pursue my dream as an author, and he took a break from his drama dreams to pursue other artistic venues.

Seasons.

God has great things in store for each of us if we'll let him have his way. Trust him. His vision of what's around the bend is never obstructed.

Follow your dreamsicles.

*Taste and see that the LORD is good;*
*blessed is the man who takes refuge in him.*
PSALM 34:8

## Scoop for Thought

God calls us to rise above our circumstances. And sometimes, he even tells us to change those circumstances. Don't be afraid to step out in faith.

Sixteen

# Pray, Lean, and Scream!

Prayer and leaning on the Lord can make all the difference in life's difficult situations. But a good scream every now and then never hurt.

*When a man has no strength, if he leans on God,*
*he becomes powerful.*
DWIGHT L. MOODY

My niece has always been big on fairy tales.

All her life she's dreamed of getting married and having kids. Whenever people asked her what she wanted to be when she grew up, she'd reply, "a wife and a mom."

So when she fell head over heels at nineteen, she figured that this first love would be her last. Her happily ever after. But after three years of dating, her boyfriend, who had told her she was "the one" for him, suddenly said he needed some "space."

What he really meant was another "S" word: *sayonara.*

Although things hadn't been that great between them for a while, the breakup still hurt. Later, as she was going through all the cards and love letters he'd written her over the years, she began to cry. Then she screamed out to God, "Why?! Why?! Why do I have to get hurt? Why couldn't I marry my first love like I'd always wanted to?"

Now, after prayer and time, she's wisely realized that life isn't a fairy tale. "God has shown me that, instead of relying on a man to fulfill my dreams, that's what he's there for," she says.

With her ex-boyfriend, a real body-conscious guy who pumped iron five days a week, my niece never felt thin enough, or pretty enough, or smart enough. Now she has a new perspective. "God loves me and accepts me as I am," she says simply. "I was created in his image, and nothing he created is ugly."

You go, sweetie!

I need to remember that myself on my bad hair, meno-
pausal mood swing days.

Recently, I attended a business dinner at an out-of-town
convention in Atlanta with some publishing colleagues.
A group of us shared a cab back to our respective hotels,
and as we pulled up to the first hotel, I reached into my
purse to get some money for the fare.

Problem was, earlier when I'd switched from my large
day purse to my smaller evening purse, I hadn't had time
to remove the essentials from my wallet. So, running late,
I just jammed my thick, bulging-at-the-seams wallet into
my slender evening purse.

Removing my too-big black wallet from my too-small
black purse in a dark cab was like trying to pull my fresh-
from-the-dryer too-tight jeans up over my too-wide hips.
While I was trying to yank my stubborn wallet from the
confines of my purse, I was at the same time trying to hold
up my end of a sparkling conversation with all my literary friends and colleagues.

Success at last!

My wallet was finally free from the stubborn clutch of
the tiny black purse. By that time, however, someone else
had already paid the full fare, so I promptly forgot about
my wallet and focused my energies on making a good
conversation impression instead.

Ten minutes later, I arrived at my destination where I
was excited to catch up with some friends I hadn't seen
in over a year. Only a couple members of our party had
arrived, my friend Becky and a new friend, Lee, whom I'd
just met earlier that day.

I joined them and ordered a soft drink. When the
waiter delivered it, I reached into my recalcitrant purse

to pay and was pleasantly surprised to open it with nary a struggle.

That's when I discovered my wallet was missing.

Blind panic. Especially since I would have to fly home the next day and wouldn't have any ID.

Becky generously paid for my drink as I retraced my steps outside to where the cab had dropped me off.

No wallet.

I asked the valet parking attendants if a wallet had been turned in.

Nope.

Using Lee's cell phone, I called another friend, Chip, from the group who'd ridden in the cab with me to see if he'd found my wallet.

Nope again.

Then Lee donned his shining armor suit and with a little crafty Sherlock Holmes sleuthing helped me figure out the name of the cab company and put in a call to report the missing wallet.

By this time, the rest of our party had arrived, looking gorgeous, including my good friend Ellie. I looked a little less than gorgeous as I was perspiring profusely from a hot flash. Ellie kindly walked me back outside to the front of the hotel, praying all the way that the Lord would reveal the location of the missing wallet to us.

Nothing.

We returned to the others, and I decided I'd better go back to my hotel so I could call Michael and have him put a stop on all our credit cards.

W-a-a-a-h-h! Then I remembered I didn't even have any money to get back to the hotel! My friends passed the hat for me, and I started to stand up to leave.

Before I left, though, Donna, another new friend I'd just met that day, said, "Wait. Let's pray first." So, we all bowed our heads in the lobby of the Ritz Hotel in Atlanta while Donna loudly and fervently prayed, "Lord, you know where Laura is, and you know where that wallet is, and we know you can bring those two together. We trust you for the outcome. Amen."

I started to leave, and Lee's cell phone rang. As he answered it, he said, "Wait. This might be for you, Laura."

I looked at him skeptically and thought *Ri-ight.* . . .

Lee began nodding and smiling into the phone, looking at me during the whole conversation. When he hung up, he did that guy thing of "YES-S-S!" where he made a fist and pulled it in to himself in exultation.

"That was Chip calling," he said. "Annette [another author friend who'd shared our cab] has your wallet."

I screamed.

> *The prayer of a righteous [wo]man is*
> *powerful and effective.*
> JAMES 5:16

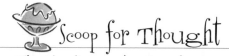 Scoop for Thought

There's a time and a place for screaming, but prayer needs no special time or place. Pray more; scream less.

# Seventeen

# Through the Rocky Road and into the Rainbow Sherbet

Laughter, healing (and a marshmallow or two)
for life's bumpy spots.
After the rain, there's always a rainbow.

*The way I see it, if you want the rainbow,*
*you gotta put up with the rain.*
DOLLY PARTON

When my friend Sally Klein O'Connor was eight years old, a dog bit her in the face.

It took a hundred stitches to sew her torn face back together. And when she returned to school—a brand-new school since her family had recently moved—the kids called her "Scarface." This to a pretty little girl who used to play the princess in the family backyard productions of fairy tale plays.

That little girl no longer felt pretty. And the children's taunts left a much deeper scar than the one on her cheek.

For years, Sally not only felt ugly, she became ugly, she now admits. "I knew how to speak ugly. I knew how to dress ugly. I knew how to act ugly. It was a real safe place to be," she said. "Ugly people aren't bothered a lot." As a teenager and young woman, Sally would dress in "anonymous" clothes—men's oversized flannel shirts, blue jeans, and high-top tennis shoes, because she was afraid of being a woman.

It was much easier being a person.

"How can you conceive of yourself as a woman when your identity is a scarface?" she asked.

But nearly twenty years after that rocky childhood road, Sally left that "safe" place of ugliness and began to heal, thanks to a new, deep, and intimate relationship with the living God. He showed her a new way to see herself, not out of her pain but out of his love. This song, written by Sally and her husband, Michael, illustrates that.

### Let Me Be Your Eyes

*Nobody ever told you you're beautiful*
*A simple solitary shining star*
*So when the world held up its mirror*
*You gladly bought the lie*
*That beauty's how you look, not who you are*

*You studied all your lines and got the part down*
*But you could never win your own applause*
*Hey don't you know by now*
*You're a diamond in My sight*
*And My love will see you through the flaws*

*When the world has you believin'*
*All its superficial lies*
*Let Me be, let Me be your eyes*
*In your heart the scars run tough and tender*
*From all the inner battles you've been through*
*So when you look to your reflection and it's hard*
*for you to see*
*Then Baby count on Me to look for you*

*I'm gonna paint a picture you can believe*
*I'm gonna teach you how to see*
*That the truest mirror of all*
*Is found in the eyes of Love*

Sally is now a singer and songwriter married to a man who calls her "Beauty." She's also the mother of two beautiful daughters, Dusty and Bonnie, and she and her songwriter husband, Michael, have a touring music ministry that brings hope and healing to the hurting.

I first met Sally when I was a reporter for a Sacramento newspaper and was assigned to cover a concert she was giving at a local church. Her songs made me—and everyone else in the audience—weep, as she shared her powerful stories that cut straight to the heart. Her music spoke volumes to me, as did the radiant beauty emanating from her as she leaned her head back in glorious abandonment and exultation to God.

Later, when I conducted a follow-up phone interview with Sally and her husband, we discovered that her husband, Michael, had known my husband, Michael, in college, but they'd lost touch over the years. In fact, her Michael had directed my Michael in a reader's theater production of a Broadway musical!

Small world.

My Michael's been acting since high school. It's his passion. But earning a living as an actor—unless you're Tom Hanks or Robert DeNiro—is not an easy task. So, my wonderfully talented husband instead holds down a "real job" during the day and acts on occasion, mainly in church productions.

---

Earning a living as an actor—
unless you're Tom Hanks or
Robert DeNiro—is not an easy task.

---

For years, we attended a huge church that put on an annual Christmas extravaganza with lots of razzle-dazzle, special effects, and a cast of hundreds. Michael was usually involved in several aspects of the production—from acting and singing to directing and making props. (I'll never forget the year I helped him paint seventy three-foot-tall wooden candy canes.)

But what he really wants to do is act. He longs to do Chekhov (which, as far as I know, isn't done in church) or at least something with a little dramatic "meat" to it.

So Michael was thrilled the year our church's music director called and told him he'd written a part especially for him for the Christmas show. He was even more thrilled when he read the script. The main character definitely had some "meat," not to mention a beautiful solo.

Michael went to the first audition and knocked 'em dead.

The "callback" audition, same thing.

But God had other plans.

The next morning, the music director gave the role to someone else. Someone with virtually no acting experience. Someone God had told him to cast.

Michael was devastated.

Finally he gets a role he can sink his teeth into. A role that's written for him. A role he loves. And it gets yanked away at the eleventh hour without warning.

Not only that; the producer asked Michael if he would direct the play and coach the actor—and the other main actors in the cast—who'd been given Michael's role.

My husband struggled mightily through this rocky road experience, and so did I. As his wife, who knew more than anyone just how much he'd set his heart on this role, I raged at the injustice of the situation. I was angry and upset that my husband had been hurt and disappointed this way.

It wasn't fair!

But Michael, who'd been praying long and hard for many weeks about the casting of this show, accepted this as God's plan. He gently defused my anger by saying, "Well, who am I to stand in the way of God? If God has handpicked someone else for the role, then who am I to argue, even if I don't understand or know the reason? What I do know is God is in control, and he has reasons we don't always see. It's not about me—or anyone—being in a role, it's about his work, which is an outreach to draw people to Christ."

But acceptance within one's mind doesn't necessarily coincide with the feelings.

In his head, Michael knew he was doing the right thing, but he was still hurt and disappointed. While the cast did not know he had waited more than ten years for a role like this one, they were all aware that something out of the norm was going on. Some feared we might even leave the church over it (something that never entered our minds), and others, that he'd drop out of the worship ministry.

So a major chunk of the first rehearsal was a time of sharing. A time of dying to self for Michael and the cast of players. Michael firmly believes this was a time of purification so that God could do his work through them and through the production.

And so, for the next several weeks, Michael directed and coached the actors. And the show went on.

And hundreds of people came to Christ.

Sure, it was a rocky road. It would have been very easy to turn back and look for a smoother path. But where would we be then?

Only by walking down God's intended road, even when it's rocky, can we get to his promised rainbow sherbet.

### Come and Follow Me

*Has the world disappointed you?*
*All your hopes and dreams fallen through*
*I'm calling you*
*Come and follow Me*

*Though your heart has cried endlessly*
*Lay your net aside, leave the sea*
*Now you're free*
*To come and follow Me*

*I promise you sunshine*
*To guide you through the pain*
*You'll see My best colors*
*Every time it rains*

*There's a rocky road up ahead*
*Drop your load and I'll be your bed*
*I'll cover you, and others who*
*Follow Me*

*Break My bread tonight when you sup*
*Drink the wine and I'll fill you up*
*Take from My cup the strength you need*
*To follow Me*

*I promise you sunshine*
*To guide you through the pain*
*You'll see My best colors*
*Every time it rains*

*Though your heart has cried endlessly*
*Lay your net aside, leave the sea*
*Now you're free*
*To come and follow Me*
(© IMPROBABLE PEOPLE MINISTRIES, MICHAEL AND SALLY O'CONNOR,
ALL RIGHTS RESERVED)

I've walked down many rocky roads I didn't want to and had my share of life's hard licks. Discovering the day after my first wedding anniversary that I had breast cancer was one of them.

But the rainbow sherbet there was that God took that difficult experience and used it to help other women going through the same thing. He took something bad and used it for good. Remembering that gives me hope and peace as I encounter other rocks—or huge, crushing boulders—in the road of life.

God promises us rainbows. All we have to do is look up to see them.

*All our difficulties are only platforms for the*
*manifestation of His grace, power, and love.*
HUDSON TAYLOR

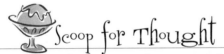 Scoop for Thought

Rocky roads are never fun or easy. But with God's abiding love and grace he'll guide us through them. We just need to follow him.

# Acknowledgments

A big scoop of thanks to everyone who shared their ice-cream stories with me: Kathy Christensen, Curt and Peggy Clark, Barb Colwell, Jan Coleman, Sara Dougherty, Bettie Eichenberg, Karen Grant, Marian Hitchings, Sheri, Kari, and Jennie Jameson, Lucille LaPoint, Pat and Ken McLatchey, Mike and Sally O'Connor, Lori Wall, and Lana Yarbrough. Although not all of them made it into the book, I really appreciate your tasty contributions!

A double scoop of thanks to my sweet nieces, Jennie and Kari, for allowing me to tell their adorable—and sometimes embarrassing—childhood stories to the whole world. A triple scoop of thanks to their mom, Sheri, for having them—and for filling in the story gaps over lunch.

Hot fudge sundae thanks to my sweet Aunt Lucille and cousins Kathy and Barb for that nostalgic walk down Goley's memory lane.

Whipped cream thanks with a cherry on top to my beloved mom for filling in the holes from my little-girl memory of Todd and the keyhole incident. And as always, thanks, Mom, for your continual support and encouragement. You're the peaches and cream.

A sorbet scoop of gratitude to my dear friends Pat and Lana, who, during our annual fall birthday tea when I was whining about writer's block, put their heads together to come up with some cute and funny stories to bail me out. I promise not to whine at next year's tea.

Hand-cranked ice-cream thanks to my country-gal writing buddy Jan, who allowed me to adapt her "Silly Goose" tale for this book.

A half-gallon of thanks to Marian Hitchings, who, along with Nessie and Angus, so graciously opened her home to me for a much-needed writing hideaway when phones and daily interruptions were about to send me over the rocky road edge.

A big Texas-sized scoop of gratitude to my sweet writing friend Annette Smith, who, although she was crunching on deadlines for *her* book, generously took the time to read some early chapters and offer feedback. Thanks too for the great ice-cream sandwich description.

Chocolate-chip-cookie-dough thanks to my "gurrl-friend" Julie Barnhill for retrieving my lost wallet story from cyberspace.

Triple chocolate thanks to Mike and Sally O'Connor and Improbable People Ministries for allowing me to use their two beautiful songs from their *Hey God, Are You Talkin' to Me?* CD. Thanks also, Sally, for allowing me to share your story.

A rainbow sherbet scoop of thanks to Twila Bennett and the dynamic duo of Karens in the publicity department: Karen Steele and Karen Van Valkenburg. Thank you for everything you do to promote my books. And, Karen V., I still owe you a big birthday dish of ice cream!

A pint of peach yogurt of thanks to my lactose-intolerant editor, Lonnie Hull DuPont, who knew how much I struggled through this book and who gently steered me in the right direction when I got off track. Your insightful comments made this a much better book. Couldn't have done it without you. Thanks for being not only the best editor but also my dear friend.

Pistachio nut thanks to my wild-and-crazy agent Chip MacGregor, who always champions my writing. Thanks for all the times you've gone above and beyond for me.

But most of all, thirty-one flavors of thanks to my Michael, who rode gallantly to the rescue when I lost my first reader Katie to a brand-new baby. (Sweet congratulations, Mark and Katie, on God's beautiful and precious gift to your family!) Honey, thank you for all those late nights of letting me read parts aloud to you, taking chapters to work to edit on your lunch hour, and even contributing some fabulous, beautifully written nuggets along the way. Now you can add writer to your list of Renaissance-man accomplishments. We make a great team, and I look forward to the day when there's a book with both our names on the cover!

**Laura Jensen Walker** is a popular speaker and breast cancer survivor who knows first-hand the healing power of laughter. She and her husband, Michael, live in Sacramento, California.

For information on having Laura Jensen Walker speak at your event, please contact Speak Up Speaker Services toll free at (888) 870-7719 or e-mail Speakupinc@aol.com. To learn more about Laura, please visit her web site at: www.laurajensenwalker.com. To write Laura, please e-mail her at Ljenwalk@aol.com or write to her at P.O. Box 601325, Sacramento, CA 95860.

"Let Me Be Your Eyes" and "Come and Follow Me" written by Michael and Sally O'Connor. Used by permission. © Copyright 1990 Improbable People Ministries. All rights reserved.

To learn more about Improbable People Ministries, please visit their web site at: www.improbablepeople.org.